The Long Search

Managing Rheumatoid Arthritis without the Use of Drugs A Personal Story

Kathryn Lausevic

www.skylark-kl.co.uk
Email: kathrynlausevic@tiscali.co.uk

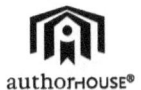

authorHOUSE®

AuthorHouse™ UK Ltd.
500 Avebury Boulevard
Central Milton Keynes, MK9 2BE
www.authorhouse.co.uk
Phone: 08001974150

First published by AuthorHouse 4/30/2010

ISBN: 978-1-4520-0221-7 (sc)

This book is printed on acid-free paper.

Dedication

To Christina, Nick and Wendy, with appreciative thanks for their love, support and friendship, which I value greatly.

To all the people who have given me support, encouragement and inspiration, with loving gratitude.

Last, but not least, to all arthritis sufferers everywhere.

It has all been a big learning process.

Contents

PART 3. SOME THEORIES ON THE CAUSES OF RHEUMATOID ARTHRITIS

INTRODUCTION

Rheumatoid arthritis is a disease which affects thousands of people. At best, it can be mild and inconvenient, affecting only a few joints, perhaps the knuckles of the hands; or it may be severe and crippling, causing the sufferer great pain, disability and stiffness. Some people have undergone many operations to try to alleviate their condition and improve mobility.

This unpleasant disease started to affect me when I was in my late forties. I was beginning to enjoy a little new-found freedom, as my children were more or less grown up, and in spite of teaching part time in a private school, I was finding more time to pursue my own interests.

This book is not aimed at any particular section of the community, but at anyone who cares to read it, especially fellow sufferers. I should like to think that some doctors may find it of interest, and hope I have not made too many medical errors, as I do not pretend to be an expert on the subject; all I can tell you is of my own experience as I tried to improve my condition, and the progress I made, by various means which some allopathic doctors might describe as "unorthodox", although it is clear that more interest is now being shown in complementary therapies, especially in diet. I can only say that my condition has improved beyond all expectation since the time I began to take responsibility for my own body, learning of its limitations and the various factors which affect it.

The book is divided into two sections. The first section of the book tells my personal story, while the second part is about holistic healing. This includes ways of self-help such as diet, exercise and other practical methods of help, followed by the spiritual, mental and emotional aspects. There is also a chapter about the possible causes of the disease.

It is not necessary to read the book in a linear fashion; some chapters may appeal to you more than others, and you may like to dig and delve! However you use the book, if you find something of interest and even help, it will have been worth my while to write it.

The orthodox medical way has been, for many years, to regard patients as "victims" of diseases, using disease-orientated language. People have been put into categories, and all with the same "label" have been treated in a similar way, commonly with drug medication, which merely suppresses the symptoms.

But diseases don't just "happen" to people. There is always a reason for one's condition.

A New Paradigm in Medicine.

Many doctors nowadays are beginning to change their attitudes to disease and methods of treatment. There is a growing awareness of a holistic way of looking at ill-health, which is "patient-centred" rather than "disease-centred."

This exciting new paradigm is concerned with the causes of disease, the reasons why a person becomes ill. It appears that irregularities in the body's biochemistry and also an impaired immune system are key factors in one's state of health.

Pioneers of the new ideas in medicine include two American doctors, Dr. Jeffrey Bland, a leading educator in biochemistry and immunology and author of the book,"The 20 Day Rejuvenation Diet Programme,"and Dr. Sidney MacDonald Baker, who specialises in the environmental and biochemical aspects of chronic health problems.

I was delighted to read Dr. Baker's book, "Detoxification and Healing", in which he declares that each patient is an individual, with a set of symptoms which show imbalances in the body. He maintains that the causes of ill-health are based on a disruption of the dynamic balance which exists between the individual and his environment; also an imbalance in the interactions between the many functions in the body.

Respecting the patient's individuality, doctors are able to look at patients' symptoms, observe signs and carry out laboratory tests, and with the use of computer technology they would be able to record all possible indications of abnormalities. There is usually more than one contributory factor in chronic conditions and this technology would enable doctors to see the whole picture. Dr. Baker calls this "Cyberhealth". Of course, these ideas come from America, and maybe it is a little idealistic to hope that it could happen in the U.K. But nothing is impossible!

Dr. Baker suggests that patients often need to change something in their lives, and the ones who do best are the ones who are prepared to do this. The changes that are needed vary with the individual.

One interesting theory is that disease (dis-ease) arises when one goes against the flow of nature, causing disharmony between mind and soul, and that it has a beneficent effect in that it brings back the personality to soul orientation, strengthening mental, emotional and physical aspects of one's being. We have to learn to listen to our body; not to do anything which goes against the harmony of its being, thereby causing stress or tension whether on a physical, mental or emotional level. Ideally one is in a state of equilibrium.

Many discoveries have been made during my search, including the importance of seemingly ordinary things like regular exercise, fresh air and relaxation; but also I have discovered the value of the use of therapies such as massage and acupuncture; fasting and herbs to cleanse the system of toxins; diet and juice therapy for energy and nutrients; vitamins and minerals; and perhaps the most surprising discovery of all, the connection with allergies, or perhaps more accurately, intolerances to certain foods substances. This of course again is connected with the balance in the body's biochemistry.

In his illuminating book, "Arthritis-The Allergy Connection," Dr. John Mansfield states:

"The concept that food allergy is an important factor in disease has advanced enormously in the past few years and more and more physicians from academic medicine are becoming actively involved in it."

The practice of Meditation has played an indispensable part in my progress and has proved itself to be a powerful aid to healing. I believe that it has a beneficial effect on the immune system, and exemplifies how the mind can radically affect the body. In particular, self-healing meditations have a dynamic effect when performed diligently and regularly.

Spiritual healing, such as that practised by the White Eagle healers or other organisations such as the National Federation of Spiritual Healers has also been a powerful aid in my progress. This form of healing can precipitate the patient's own healing process to begin to manifest.

An invaluable source of help has been the Arthritic Association, to whom I am indebted for their wonderful knowledge of arthritis problems and how to alleviate them. Their advice and dietary guidance, as well as their herbal preparations, have greatly contributed to my improvement.

This book is the story of a search and a journey. The search, on a physical level, was, and is for the possible causes of the disease, so that they could be dealt with to the best of my ability. This search, if not for an absolute cure has brought about a compromise which enables me to manage myself and my life in the best possible way, at the present time. Of course there is always more to learn!

The journey is not one in time or space, but has been -and indeed continues to be- an inner journey of learning how to deal with experiences, with whatever happens in my life. It involves going through processes which change and transform attitudes, not only to the seemingly "painful" experiences, but also to the people around me and to my environment, both in the immediate surroundings and in the greater world of which I am a part.

There are many difficulties and challenges in everyone's lives; just in day-to-day living we encounter what we think of as "problems". This is particularly so in a disease like arthritis, where dozens of difficulties arise each day, connected with actions which are trivial to an able, fit person. An example of this might be putting on one's coat, or shoes, or, my favourite pastime, dropping things on the floor! These challenges occur so frequently that if we meet them with frustration and a negative attitude, life would become unbearable; we would become impossible to ourselves and those around us, so it is really a matter of self-preservation. We have to teach ourselves to smile at difficulties, seeing each one as a little personal test and an opportunity for personal growth, perhaps change even, thereby becoming stronger, more integrated as a person, and certainly happier. Because of this, we are able to welcome each challenge, even to give thanks for it, because of the gifts it brings to us.

I also believe that we are presented with the lessons we need to learn in life. Elisabeth Kubler Ross, well-known author and researcher on Death, Dying and other spiritual matters declared,

"Humankind learns much faster through adversity. If everything is easy and no obstacle is in our way, we never learn anything."

There are many things we can learn from arthritis. Apart from finding out the physical ways of how to manage ourselves and improve our condition, we can gain attributes such as patience, tolerance, inventiveness, and appreciation of others. We can also learn to accept ourselves and our limitations with courage, patience, a sense of humour and equanimity.

PROLOGUE

It was Boxing Day,1989. My eyes opened to the dim light outlining the curtain. Taking a few deep breaths, I tried to stretch my arms and legs, but found I could not move. I tried again. Pain and stiffness suffused my body.

I waited a few moments for signs of movement from the other bed in the room, but could only hear my husband's gentle breathing. But I needed to attend to the "call of nature."

"Alex!" He stirred. I repeated his name; he moved. "Yes?"

"Alex, I can't move! Please can you massage my arms and legs a bit?" During the past few years he had often helped by massaging my arms and shoulders, when the pain had been particularly tiresome.

After some moments of re-orientating himself he came and sat on the bed, then gently began to rub my arms and legs.

Soon I was able to sit up, gingerly and very slowly, then to stand, and after some moments, to shuffle to the bathroom.

All that day, I stayed in the flat, resting, and only just managing to walk occasionally to the kitchen or the bathroom.

We were spending Christmas with our daughter, Christina, who was living near Heidelberg,Germany, teaching English. We had arrived three days earlier and had already visited the beautiful city, with its wide river, admiring the ancient buildings, and spending some time in the Christmas Market.

The previous day, we had visited a restaurant for Christmas dinner. There were six of us in the party: my husband Alex, our son Nick, daughter Christina, her boyfriend John, also his brother Peter, who had accompanied us on the visit, and was partially disabled owing to a stroke he had suffered some fourteen years previously, and myself. We had brought a wheelchair over from with us from England, and Peter and I took turns in using it, as we both had limited walking ability.

The restaurant was full of relaxed people, bursting with bonhomie, and the atmosphere was conducive to eating "well."

The meal began with a creamy soup, I remember, then for the main course I chose trout, cooked in a rich, creamy sauce, with vegetables. To finish the meal I opted for ice-cream accompanied by hot blackberry sauce. Delicious!

Now, the next morning, I was regretting having devoured so much rich food. I knew from experience that it was affecting me. In addition to this, my weight had gradually crept up over recent years; now it was about ten and a half stones, far too much for my height of five feet two inches!

After the fright I had experienced on Boxing Day morning, I felt that if I continued like this, I would be confined to a wheelchair in the not-too-distant future.

Something needed to be done! And SOON!

PART 1.
THE STORY

CHAPTER 1.
THE START OF IT ALL

Rheumatoid arthritis may cause only a mild discomfort. At the other extreme, it can devastate one's life. Apart from the pain, it can cause disability and complete dependence on others. Most sufferers come somewhere between these two polarities. Yet you often see them smiling through their pain and discomfort.

People are wonderful; some of them have a sort of self-esteem which enables them to be brave, especially when they are with others, but when they are alone it can be a vastly different story. That is when despair may well up inside.

I will not describe the physical pain in too much detail. It was written somewhere that it is like "toothache all over the body", and this seems an apt description, especially on a "bad" day. If you have ever suffered from tennis elbow, imagine that you have it in every one of your joints. You can imagine what it would be like if you knocked against something!

Although the pain was bad enough, it didn't bother me as much as the lack of mobility, which was increasing over the months and years.

The first signs of rheumatoid arthritis had shown themselves in 1984. Six years previously I had taken part in a sponsored walk which had left me with some pain in the left hip, and a decided limp; after X-rays I was told by the consultant that at some future date I would probably need a hip replacement.

But rheumatoid arthritis was something different.

The first signs of trouble surfaced during the spring of 1984, when some friends and I were visiting Glasgow, principally to see an Art and Craft Exhibition, the Burrell Collection. We enjoyed the week-end, but on the return journey, sitting in the car, I found that I could hardly move my head, due to stiffness and pain in the neck. We put this down to sitting in a draught, and after several weeks it had virtually disappeared.

At the time, I had a part-time job teaching at a girls' private school and really enjoyed my work. One lunchtime, I was standing on the landing at school, watching a group of girls practising using the computers, admiring their skill and dexterity. Turning to leave, however, I found I could hardly walk, due to sudden pain in the hip and groin. One minute I seemed to be all right, the next moment I could hardly move. What on earth was happening?

After a few minutes I was able to walk slowly to the classroom and resume my normal lessons, but the experience had been deeply disturbing.

To my dismay, the pain in the hips and groin continued intermittently throughout the summer. Then, one morning in October, I awoke to find that my hands were terribly swollen and painful. Whatever next? I decided that a trip to the doctor's was advisable.

My G.P. diagnosed suspected rheumatoid arthritis and sent me to the hospital to see a rheumatologist, who suggested that I should be admitted to the local hospital for three weeks. I wondered what the reasons were for being admitted, and the doctor explained this to me.

The reasons for admittance to hospital are mainly, to confirm the diagnosis by blood tests and other factors; to begin drug therapy, and to teach the patient how to manage the disease and also how to cope with everyday difficulties, through the means of physiotherapy and occupational therapy. So I agreed to be admitted.

In the hospital ward were about twenty-four beds, all of which were occupied by people with arthritis in varying degrees of severity. One lady had only the knuckles affected, and was receiving cortisone injections; another woman spent most of the time in bed, afraid to stand and walk as her knees gave way beneath her. The nurses spent a great deal of time trying to get her walking.

Each day we attended the physiotherapy department, where we were taught certain exercises which should be practised on a daily basis. (These were taped for us if we supplied a cassette.) The exercises are extremely important for mobility and to avoid instability in the joints. They also strengthen the muscles and increase stamina, thereby keeping you as fit as possible. I still use the tape nearly every morning. If I miss more than two mornings the effects are tangible; as well as increased stiffness and greater difficulty of movement, I feel more lethargic, with a noticeable decrease in energy. So performing the exercises is a priority.

In the occupational therapy room, as well as learning useful activities to exercise our hands, we learned all about the many and various aids and gadgets which are available for use at home. There are plenty of these aids and some of them have become absolutely indispensable to me, such as the handy potato peeler, a metal one shaped like a "U" with a bar across; the special gadget for opening lids on jars, and some well-designed, convenient kitchen taps with levers.

The drugs which I was prescribed at the time were Sulphasalazene and Voltarol. The Voltarol is an anti- inflammatory-cum-painkilling drug and I was to take one each day. Sulphasalazene is a "disease-modifying" drug, also used in the treatment of ulcerative colitis.

It was December, and apart from physiotherapy in the mornings, and occupational therapy in the afternoons, (where I painstakingly produced a macrame plant holder which I gave my mother-in-law for Christmas,) I remember that a lot of my time was spent in selling tickets for the Christmas raffle! I was quite glad to do this as it gave me a chance to talk to the other patients, as well as being a useful, positive thing to do.

As it was Christmastime, the nurses and physiotherapists had arranged an entertainment for some of the patients. The impersonal hospital room had been decorated with garlands and balloons for the occasion, and was packed with patients, a great number of whom were in wheelchairs, of all ages, both sexes and varying moods. The brave attempts of the "entertainers" brought peals of laughter from most of the audience, but for me the merriment was mingled with tears, I was so moved by it all. It was an indescribable experience.

I returned home from hospital in time for Christmas, and was glad of the help offered by my family, especially in cooking the Christmas dinner! Both my husband and son, who lived at home at the time, are now competent cooks. Over the years they even learned to enjoy cooking, which was just as well, as sometimes I was in too much pain to prepare a meal or even to perform ordinary household tasks. They became accustomed to doing all sorts of jobs in the house, in a practical, unselfish way, as is often the case where one member is not as able as he or she might be.

During the next two years my condition gradually deteriorated, although occasionally I would have a "good" day, with little pain. In 1986 the hips became more of a problem, and by July I was using crutches.

On seeing the rheumatologist at the hospital in the autumn, we discussed the possibility of a hip-replacement operation, but he thought it was unlikely that the consultant would agree to it because of my age, which was fifty-one at the time. Surgeons were reluctant to perform hip-replacements on people under sixty; this was because, after some years, the operation had to be repeated as the new "joints" gradually loosened, due to the deterioration of the cement that was used.

By November, 1986, the pain in my right hip and also the right knee was so acute that I was spending some days mostly in bed. I could hardly walk, and if I went downstairs there was tremendous difficulty in climbing up again. I remember standing at the bottom of the staircase, trying to muster the strength to ascend this upward climb, which to me looked like Everest!

In addition to these problems, there was considerable pain in the shoulders, neck, and muscles in the upper arms, partly due, no doubt, to having to use the crutches. I am describing this to give you some idea of my condition at that time.

In December an appointment was made for me to see the surgeon, Mr. Getty. In his consulting room he asked me to walk across the room without the aid of the crutches. I could not do it! He then arranged for X-rays to be taken. After studying these he decided to perform a bi-lateral hip replacement operation, which caused me some surprise. "Do you mean both together?" I asked inanely. I had never heard of it. But he assured me that it was standard practice.

So, in January, 1987, I had the operation, in a private clinic, as we were members of an insurance scheme. Both before the operation and afterwards I felt very calm, spending some time practising deep breathing exercises to relax myself as much as possible. I had learned these in Yoga classes which I had attended over the years and really enjoyed. Now I was making good use of what I had learned.

After the operation I made good progress. This was partly due to having practised the daily exercises taught to me by the physiotherapist prior to the operation, and for which I was extremely grateful. The health service is excellent in some ways! We should not underestimate its value.

I spent seventeen days in the clinic. Before I left I was able to walk up and down the stairs and also to take a bath. This is not as simple as it sounds, as you need considerable help in getting in and out of the bath, at least at first.

So, with renewed hope and optimism, I returned home, although I now know it is best to have "no expectations!"

Several weeks after my return, some problems began to arise. One difficulty was that I had been instructed by the surgeon to sleep on my back for three months; this caused some soreness in places which were pressing on the bed, especially the buttocks and heels. I tried sleeping on a sheepskin but this made me very hot. I was also experiencing a great deal of pain in the shoulders, elbows and arm muscles, probably through using the crutches. In addition to this the last three fingers of the left hand had become numb and "tingly." I remember the difficulty of lifting the cup of water which was kept by my bed, during the night when I needed a drink; the arms were so stiff and painful I could hardly lift the cup. This problem was eased somewhat with the help of massage, and some useful exercises, for instance shrugging the shoulders. Yoga exercises were also helpful, especially in relaxing the muscles.

In spite of these challenges, three months after the operation I was able to walk to the local shops, a distance of about two hundred yards, with the aid of the crutches of course. The first time I did this a friend accompanied me in her car, to check that I was all right. Previously I had walked as far as the house next door but one. The people who lived there were called "Mountain." So when my husband, Alex, came home from work I told him I had walked as far as the Mountains and back!

Then, some good news! When I saw the surgeon for the three-monthly check-up, he gave me permission to a) drive, b) swim, and, best of all, to lie on my side in bed. This was bliss indeed, and felt absolutely wonderful! Also in May, I was able to get out of the bath by myself. Things were looking up!

During the rest of that year the pain fluctuated considerably; during the "bad" periods the Voltarol was increased to two a day, as the rheumatologist had advised.

This chapter sounds very "one-sided" as it merely describes my physical state at this time. However, many other events were happening in my life, some of them very meaningful, especially connected with the spiritual side, and I shall mention this in a later chapter.

When I felt well enough and physically able, I attended the yoga class, as the feeling of serenity and well-being derived from it was extremely important and beneficial. Yoga works on the mind and spirit, as well as on the physical body. As I have already said, I had practised it for many years and really appreciated the classes.

In January 1988 our yoga teachers David and Enid started to teach us more about methods of healing, and healing in general. Enid was talking about the nature of disease, and told us that one of the underlying factors in arthritis was thought by certain people to be <u>pride</u>.

This gave me food for thought, and I remembered the times that I had been "hurt" in some way, by some word or action that someone had said or done, probably thoughtlessly; I realised that it was my pride that was hurt. This was a fault in me, and something to work on, if I could. Another manifestation of pride is too much self-reliance, which shows itself in trying to perform tasks which risk harming the joints, rather than asking for help if it is available. This causes more suffering and in the long run is counter-productive. This was something of which I was often guilty, being unwilling to bother people if I could manage the task by myself, but if it was harming my body I realised that I should ask for help. So it was something I needed to learn.

It was a year since the hip operation and the consultant was pleased with me, although he advised me to lose a stone in weight. However he was not very pleased when I told him I had climbed up ninety-two steps on holiday! This was on the island in the middle of Lake Bled, in Slovenia, and I had been very pleased with myself on reaching the top, to admire the lovely view.

Mr.Getty's reaction to this news was "Never do that again!"

From my yoga training, I found that meditation and deep breathing were of immense benefit, giving a wonderful feeling of peace and calmness. Sometimes if I could not sleep because of discomfort, I would breathe deeply, pausing between breaths and make my mind a blank. This is a wonderful sleep-inducer!

Sometimes I would experience beautiful and inspiring dreams, which filled me with wonder and gave me great encouragement.

A typical one came in March 1988. I dreamed that Alex and I were walking in the suburbs of a town, which I did not recognise, when we arrived at a very steep hill; in fact it was so steep that it would have been impossible to climb up in the usual way. But in the dream we held hands and just sort of - well, floated up, so, so easily. I felt that I was being helped up the formidable slope, not only by Alex on my left, but by some unseen force on the right side. It was a strange yet wonderful feeling.

Dreams like this came reassuringly frequently at this time and I realised they were symbolic of the problems I was having to face in everyday life, for example the metaphor of climbing a steep slope. But in my mind I had a strong conviction that I was receiving help on an unseen level. This gave me great comfort and a certain courage, without which I cannot imagine how I would have felt.

During May of the same year the arthritis began to make itself felt in the spine. I was also having problems with the right hip, in addition to the "usual" places, such as the arms and neck. The back pain often kept me awake. One day I read an article in "Stella Polaris," the magazine of the White Eagle Church. The subject was "Suffering, and the causes of it." The writer put forward the theory that the soul, before it reincarnates, often chooses to serve God by suffering during its life on Earth, partly as an example to help others. Of course you might say, why does anyone have to suffer at all? and this is a very deep subject.

Anyway, the point of view expressed in the article appealed to me, and I felt that if this was the reason why I had this painful disease, then perhaps it was a privilege to serve in this way, and I should be glad of the opportunity to manifest a Higher purpose through me.

So I prayed that I would be worthy of it, and be given the strength to be a "shining light!" And I was going to need that strength.

During the next few months the general pain had worsened, to the point of often having to spend complete days in bed, as movement was so difficult. The wrists and ankles were now affected, also the pain in the back and shoulders was becoming more widespread. Even the jaw did not escape! It was frequently difficult to chew my food, and opening my mouth wide was so painful that I was concerned that I would not be able to have any dental treatment!

A packet of frozen peas placed on the shoulder or on other painful places helped to relieve the pain of the inflammation to some extent. The peas were kept in the freezer for just this purpose; fortunately no-one ever tried to prepare them for a meal! In any case, they had been removed and returned to the freezer so many times that they were all congealed together!

I was interested in trying to discover the reasons for my illness, so towards the end of November I booked a hypnotherapy session. It is thought, in some circles, that certain diseases are often rooted in childhood experiences, and I thought and hoped to throw some light on the subject.

Catherine, the hypnotherapist, was a young woman in her thirties. At the first session, I lay on a couch while she spoke in her gentle voice, asking me to relax each part of the body in turn, to achieve a state of deep relaxation. I began to feel really comfortable and relaxed, euphoric even. When I was completely relaxed Catherine began to encourage me to talk about certain incidents in my life, and about my childhood recollections. I talked for more than one hour. But afterwards, for the whole evening and night, I had renewed pain everywhere in my body. I felt as though I had been run over by a steam-roller! This, I thought, could only be connected with recollecting some painful events in my past experiences, and proved, once again, how powerful is the mind!

A nice little demonstration of the power of the mind had been given to us during a yoga session, some years previously. Enid had asked us to visualise a large, juicy lemon, then to take a knife and cut it into two halves. Then she asked for our reactions. All of us had "watering" mouths, almost as though we could taste the sourness of the lemon!

Anyway, to return to the aftermath of the hypnotherapy session. The following day, Thursday, found me still crying with pain and emotion. I felt as though I was disintegrating, physically and emotionally.

By the following week-end I felt a little better, but was concerned about the effect the pain was having on my joints. On telephoning the hypnotherapist, she suggested that I talk to my G.P., so I made an appointment.

The doctor, a lady, reacted to my tale of woe with kindness and understanding, stating that in her opinion there would be no detrimental effects on the joints. In fact she was extremely reassuring, and gave me her wholehearted support, saying, "We don't pretend to have the answers to everything."

Because of the after-effects of the first visit to the hypno-therapist I wasn't particularly looking forward to repeating the experience, but decided to attend for the second session with an open mind.

In fact, both the second and third sessions were quite helpful. Again I talked about my childhood and more recent experiences, releasing some tension in crying. Afterwards the feeling of relaxation lasted for the whole evening; indeed, after the third visit I felt much "lighter" and more energetic, so much so that the following day saw me performing a great number of household tasks, - polishing, washing ornaments, cleaning woodwork and so on, jobs which were normally neglected! I also baked some cheese scones in preparation for the proposed visit of some people from the L.I.F.E. Foundation, a holistic therapy organisation, who were due to visit Sheffield the following week-end. Dr.Patel, or "Manny" as we affectionately called him, was coming to give a talk on The Nature and Causes of Disease. I was certainly looking forward to it.

CHAPTER 2.
REVELATIONS

Little did I suspect, as I prepared to go to my dear friend Dorothy's house, that this particular evening, November 25th., 1988, would not only be extremely memorable for me, but that it would herald the beginning of a change in my life, a sort of "transformation" in myself and my ways of thinking.

On arriving at Dorothy's beautiful bungalow, where we normally held our yoga group in the spacious attic room, I saw that the large, comfortable lounge was filled with chairs in readiness for the lecture. After taking off my coat I went to help prepare refreshments in the kitchen, so was rather late in entering the room. When I eventually went in, the room appeared to be crammed full of people and there seemed to be no available spare seat. However, a friend, Ruth, kindly found me a chair, but it was a hard, wooden one, and I knew that I wouldn't be able to sit on it for the whole evening. Then my eye caught sight of an empty arm-chair, right at the front! Dr.Patel (Manny), who was already prepared to begin the talk, indicated that I should sit there, which I did and found it perfect!

Afterwards, I realised that if I had sat further back I would not have been able to see or hear so well; it was a slide-show and I had an excellent view.

Dr. Patel began the lecture, showing slides to illustrate the points he was making. The pictures were varied and entertaining, including some attractive ones of natural subjects:- many-coloured flowers, bright butterflies, tranquil views of the countryside and so on. Others contained information, and one of these held me transfixed. It was about early childhood.

Manny explained that if a child suffers from a lack of emotional love, or there is a sense of stress or tension in the atmosphere surrounding him/her, problems can start to occur which are potentially far-reaching, affecting the whole future of the child. The situation begins to have an effect when the child reaches the age of about seven years.

If a child is living in an inharmonious environment, or feels unloved for any reason he/she starts to behave in a way which is alien to his true nature. He starts to act in a way which he thinks is expected of him, so as to conform and earn love and approval from his parents, in order to be accepted. This rigid behaviour is a suppression of his natural responses and spontaneity.

Sometimes there is an incident which is the "last straw," and the child represses all freedom of action or word. Because the child is behaving in a way which is not natural to him, tension begins to occur. Over the years, this tension becomes a habit and may last a very long time, sometimes even a lifetime.

Now, stress and strain over a long period of time causes chemical changes in the body, which lead to a breakdown in the immune system. Manny explained that this, in turn, can lead to the onset of one of many diseases, including cancer, diabetes, multiple sclerosis, heart problems and rheumatoid arthritis!

As though a light had been switched on in my mind, I realised that this all applied to me! A piece of the jig-saw was being put into place.

Since early childhood I had been riddled with tension. The atmosphere in our house was uncomfortable, to say the least, and this had an effect on both my sister, three years older than I, and myself. The tension was the "norm" for us as we grew into adolescence, becoming ingrained in our bodies and our personalities, preventing us from expressing ourselves freely, or being in any way relaxed at home. Only since I began to practise yoga techniques have I learned how to be more relaxed, but this was done consciously, helped by the invaluable breathing techniques; it had not become part of my being until comparatively recently.

At this period of my life, however, the feeling that I was on the verge of a crisis of some sort was always present in my mind; I seemed to be walking on a "knife edge," as it were.

The tension had begun almost as far back as I could remember. I am not blaming anyone; it was just how things were. I do not wish to go into the reasons for this in detail as they are not relevant, except to say that the relationship between my parents was not an easy one; my mother suffered from poor health and my father had his own problems. The atmosphere at home, for most of the time, was an extremely fraught one, with long, tense silences.

Often I would go to the house of a friend, where the people laughed and talked easily together. This was a revelation to me, and I felt myself "unbend" a little. I didn't realise it at the time but all the girls I chose as friends were relaxed people, ones with whom I could often share fun and laughter.

Both my sister and I rebelled to some extent. We started "going out" with boys from an early age, and I remember once playing truant, which gave me a wonderful feeling of freedom. My friend, Janet and I went to Nottingham on the 'bus (we lived at Mansfield, a distance of about fourteen miles). After purchasing two "half-return" tickets we had only three-and-a-half pence between us, which we spent on sweets. Some of the time, I remember, was spent in trying on hats of all shapes and colours in C & A's Department store!

We hear a lot about drugs nowadays in connection with young people. Why do they often turn to drugs, or alcohol, or smoke excessively? My experience has caused me to think that one of the reasons could be STRESS, possibly caused by trauma in childhood. I am not suggesting that this is always the case, but some young people have such deep-down tension ingrained into them due to suppression of real feelings in childhood, or other childhood problems that they will do almost <u>anything</u> to have that relaxed feeling. I am not condoning their behaviour, just trying to understand it.

Now, Dr. Patel's words reminded me that most of the arthritis sufferers I had met seemed to be "nice" people; I had sometimes wondered why. Now I realised that they may have learned this behaviour during a difficult childhood, in order to please their loved ones and gain approval and affection, to the detriment of their own natural urges and inclinations, which became suppressed, turning inwards, eventually to harm their bodies.

However, back to the talk. Manny explained that, to combat tension and stress there are several practices which are very helpful. Yoga, relaxation techniques and meditation were mentioned, also doing things which one enjoys, such as pursuing an interesting or absorbing hobby or pastime. A man in the U.S.A. who had cancer had shut himself up in a room to watch old comedy films, and had made himself better by laughing!

Why does suppression of feelings have this effect?

When we are relaxed our immune system is able to work as it should. This happens when we have peace of mind, and feel in harmony with ourselves, with those around us, and with our environment. When we are in this state of well-being, certain physiological effects take place in our bodies. The endocrine system produces substances, certain hormones which act like drugs, which have a calming effect on mind and body. A strong immune system protects us from all kinds of ills, harmful bacteria, viruses - indeed infections of all kinds, as well as serious illnesses such as cancer and other diseases. But there is a "holistic " effect in that we enter into a state of equilibrium, a healing state if you like.

Any unrelieved stress or tension caused, for instance, by the suppression of feelings, initiates the release in the body of stress-related hormones which are connected with the onset of certain diseases.

In order to have real "peace of mind" we need to dispose of any feelings which can harm us, such as resentment, bearing grudges, judging or criticising people, anger or any feelings of dissatisfaction with others or with our lives. Of course we all have problems, but it is our *attitude* to these which makes all the difference. There is a wonderful prayer, attributed to Saint Francis, which says, "God, grant me the serenity to accept the things I cannot change, courage to change the things I can, and wisdom to know the difference."

Thinking about all these discoveries began a sort of transformation for me. At first the tension was released in tears. I would go into the bathroom, close the door, immerse myself in a warm bath, think about some traumatic event from the past and, with the radio or a cassette playing, could cry quite freely and noisily, with no-one to hear! I would think about the people who helped to shape my childhood and, with a new awareness, seem to understand them for the first time. With understanding came compassion and complete forgiveness. The result was that I began to feel more relaxed than I ever remembered feeling, since I was a small child. The sensation of release was indescribable.

After one of these sessions I noticed that the physical pain in the joints and muscles had decreased. The more tension I released, the better I felt physically!

At my next hypnotherapy session I told Catherine, the hypnotherapist about my "revelation" and that I had been releasing long-standing tensions, also that I no longer seemed to need to take sleeping tablets or paracetamol, which had been a constant "prop." In addition I had reduced the amount of arthritis drugs, as I no longer needed them so often. Catherine assured me that the healing process would continue, saying that I did not need to see her again, at least for the time being. The only advice she gave me was to be careful with my diet.

Soon after this, at the beginning of December, I decided - perhaps rashly, to stop taking drugs altogether, as an experiment. I had recently read a magazine article which described how drugs can pollute the body, not really improving the basic condition but merely suppressing the symptoms. In fact, it was stated that taken over a long period of time, they can actually make the condition considerably worse. So feeling so much better in the body, I optimistically decided to try to manage without them!

* * * * * *

Since the "magic" week-end of Dr.Patel's visit, which initiated a sort of transformation in me caused by the revelations of the lecture and the discoveries I had made, I found that strange and wonderful things were happening. For one thing, my intuition became more acute; for instance if I telephoned a friend I invariably knew if he/she was going to answer or not, while it was ringing. If I could not visualise the person it meant that they were not there. Another example is that sometimes in the morning, before I came downstairs, I would have a strong feeling that there was a letter from Tina, my daughter, and sure enough, lying on the mat, there it would be!

My powers of appreciation seemed to be increased; the colours and shapes of flowers, for instance, seemed incredibly beautiful; music was (and still is) a never-ending source of wonder and joy.

Another noticeable indication of the difference in me was that *words* held much more meaning and I began to realise how important they are. They have tremendous power which can be used for good or ill. They can be used to heal or to wound. In addition to this, everything a person says tells us something about that person; all we have to do is *listen*.

Early one morning, looking through the bedroom window, I could see dark clouds scudding across the sky, which was brightening on the horizon, but in the darkest part, higher up, were Venus, shining brightly, and a crescent moon. It was so beautiful that it moved me to tears.

I kept doing absent-minded things, for example, one morning I found the bread in the fridge, frozen solid!

The pervading feeling at this time was that all this had been part of some wondrous PLAN for me, and I felt unbelievably privileged, with a deep, inner joy.

In spite of these wonderful happenings, I was having some misgivings concerning my decision to stop taking the drugs, as by the middle of January, 1989 I was in a great deal of discomfort, about six weeks after I had taken the last dose. A result of this was that I was obliged to spend an increasing amount of time in bed. Undecided what to do, after several days of severe pain I made up my mind to write to the rheumatologist for advice, and a week or so later, with reluctance I resumed taking the sulphasalazine. There seemed to be no alternative, as I was concerned about the possibility of harm to my joints if I continued as I was.

An adverse effect of this set-back was manifested in increased immobility due to inactivity. During the winter I had neglected to do the arthritis exercises as often as I should, but a friend with R.A. reminded me that when we were in hospital, everyone had to perform the exercises every day, even the patients suffering from "flare-ups." So I began doing them again in earnest, in spite of extremely painful and inflamed knees; the beneficial effects showed themselves almost instantly, especially in the arms and shoulders.

Resting in bed, albeit enforced, brought compensations of all kinds. I had "Spiritual" magazines to read, which were a wonderful help and inspiration; also I spent considerable time listening to music, especially my cassette tapes of relaxing, ambient, gentle music, as well as a good deal of piano music by Chopin, one of my favourites. I also meditated and sent love and light to everyone I knew who had a problem, (and who doesn't?) as well as to suffering people in the world at large, to animals, and to the Earth itself. All of this helped to put my own problems into perspective. When I felt a little disillusioned with my lack of physical progress, the peace and meditation helped to restore my spirits; another enormous help was the wonderful Yoga breathing, as always.

Sometimes people came to visit - close friends and relatives who cheered me with their loving thoughtfulness.

One morning, I was thinking how difficult I found physical resistance to my body, for instance struggling with the bedclothes, switching on tight taps and so on, and wondered if it was symbolic of my attitude to resistance in my life, which would often go differently from how I would wish. So my lesson, it appeared, was to learn how to cope with feelings of frustration by being more tranquil. Then I thought this should apply to all strong emotions - fear, excitement, anger and so on; they should be treated in the same way, so that I could detach myself from them as much as possible, and just flow with everything. This was (and is) an extremely difficult lesson for me to learn, and an ongoing process, as I have always had strong feelings about things, but I had to make the attempt, with the help of yoga, meditation, relaxation and the Inner Spirit. This gave me a personal goal to aim for, and in the mornings I would be up before the sun, light a candle and meditate; this gave me a feeling of harmony and order, inspiration and much comfort. Other sources of inspiration came from the books I was reading.

Some books which helped me during this period include "Tao - The Watercourse Way," by Alan Watts, and a beautiful book by Frederick Franck entitled "The Book of Angelus Silesius," who was a 17th. century Zen poet. These books are full of inspiration and knowledge about the attributes we need to learn to attain mastery of ourselves; about equanimity - not forcing things, and being calm under all conditions. During difficult times I could remind myself of the beautiful examples given in the books.

By the end of March I began to feel somewhat better, even starting to have comparatively "good" days. Of course, I had resumed taking the drugs by this time. Now I had to be careful not to "overdo" things, which would strain the joints and aggravate the problem once more.

However, another problem began to arise in that my response to the medication was fluctuating. In spite of the positive influences in my life the physical problems became more acute, and by July, 1989 the strongest of the drugs I was taking had appeared to lose its effect, as sometimes happens in drug therapy.

A visit to the rheumatology department resulted in my commencing a course of gold injections, one per week to begin with, which seemed to help at first, but by the following Christmas my condition had deteriorated to the extent of being unable to walk more than a short distance, due to pain and stiffness. In the evenings there were "tingling" sensations all over my body, so I took myself off to bed, sometimes as early as 7p.m.

Alex, Nick and I decided to spend Christmas in Heidelberg with Tina, our daughter. We took a hired wheelchair with us; this was useful not only for myself, but also for Peter, Tina's boyfriend's brother, who accompanied us; he had walking difficulties owing to a stroke he had suffered some years previously.

As I mentioned in the prologue, we celebrated Christmas by visiting a restaurant for lunch, which for me, consisted of some extremely "rich" food, including a creamy soup, trout accompanied by a cream sauce and vegetables, then ice-cream - my favourite, with blackberry sauce. What a feast!

After this gourmet food, I found, on waking the next morning, that I could not move at all! Alex had to massage my legs before I could get out of bed.

I began to realise that if I didn't do something drastic soon, I would probably end up being completely dependent on others, for me, a horrifying thought. I knew a woman like this, completely unable to walk. As well as looking after her in the daytime, her husband had to get up every two hours in the night to turn her. What a prospect!

Apart from the pain and stiffness in the joints and muscles at this time, other related problems included irritation of the eyes, a sore tongue, and persistent thrush which I was told was a symptom of candida; also I had a tender area on the top of my head which often ached, and nodes on the backs of my wrists, but these did not bother me too much as they were not normally painful.

During the few remaining days of our holiday in Germany, my mind kept returning to two books which had been lent to me by a friend. One was about a treatment for many diseases, called the Gerson Therapy. This therapy could be used even for cancer patients, and basically involved cleansing the whole body until it was free from toxins, and following a particular diet. The method advocated consuming vegetable juices made on a juice machine, taking enemas and following the diet, which mainly consisted of salads and raw vegetables. It seemed rather extreme, but I felt that drastic measures were needed.

The other book which seemed to be pointing me in a particular direction was an Essene book, "The Gospel of Peace of Jesus Christ." This described how Jesus gave advice on the healing of diseases. Again, this was done by cleansing the body, inside and out; by fasting and by prayer.

"The body is the temple of the spirit, and the spirit is the temple of God. Purify, therefore, the temple, that the Lord of the temple may dwell therein and occupy a place that is worthy of him."

- The Gospel of Peace of Jesus Christ.

Another cleansing agent was fresh air - "Seek the fresh air of the forest and of the fields; breathe long and deeply, that the angel of air may be brought within you."

After that, the healing power of water was indicated, both externally - washing the body all over, and also internally, in taking enemas to cleanse the system.

"So I tell you truly, the angel of water shall cast out of your body all uncleannesses which defiled it without and within, so that you may become as pure as the river's foam sporting in the sunlight."

- The Gospel of Peace of Jesus Christ.

I decided to take the plunge!

CHAPTER 3.
THE THERAPY

Although I had previously tried various therapies and diets, I had not attempted anything like this before, a process of cleansing the body by removing toxins from the organs and intestines, in fact from the bloodstream and also from the tissues, - a system of whole internal cleansing.

Later, after I joined the Arthritic Association, I was to discover that their wonderful Detox tablets, taken once a week, before and during a fast, did this job on a steady, regular basis; but for now, I was willing and even eager to begin the Gerson therapy I had been reading about.

Arnold Ehret, who wrote, "The Mucousless Diet Healing System," states that the average person has as much as ten pounds of uneliminated material in the bowel continually, poisoning the bloodstream and the entire system. He declares that every sick person has a more or less mucous-clogged system, from undigested, unnatural food substances, accumulated since childhood.

I wanted to be clean inside as well as outside!

In the 1930's and 40's Dr.Max Gerson found that in all chronic degenerative diseases the patient suffers from severe nutritional deficiencies and also from toxaemia caused by accumulated waste materials and poisons from the environment and from food, especially from additives, pesticides and colourings. Nowadays we can add preservatives to this list. Many people are not aware of the extent to which these are used, not only to add shelf-life to the food, but also to make it appear more attractive to the purchaser. The appearance of organically-grown food, by contrast, is not so tempting to the average buyer, but of course nutrition-wise it is far superior, as well as being relatively free from chemicals and additives.

Dr.Gerson presented his therapy as a treatment specifically for cancer in his book: "A Cancer Therapy- Results of Fifty Cases," because this condition is the most destructive and poisonous to the human body.

The aim of the therapy is to restore the body's healing mechanism, and the function of its organs; also to support the maintenance of health. It follows that the same therapy would have these effects in other chronic conditions, such as arthritis. There is in fact a chapter in Dr. Gerson's book dealing especially with this, written by his daughter, Charlotte Gerson Straus.

Dr.Gerson found that in all chronic diseases there was a loss of potassium at the outset of the disease. Potassium, an alkali, is essential for the body to function properly, as it should. The best way to take potassium is through consuming fresh fruit and juices, so this is a crucial part of the therapy. At the same time, the body needs to be cleansed of all unwanted substances, accumulated over the years. This detoxification process is carried out mainly by means of taking coffee enemas; Dr.Gerson also advocated taking special supplements to help to regenerate the liver.

In restoring the body's functions, Dr. Gerson maintained that the body's own healing mechanism would then take over. Arthritic lumps and swellings would disappear;

moreover diseased bone would become denser and stronger. It sounded promising!

Drugs are pollutants to the body and it is advised that these should be discontinued at the start of the therapy, as the purpose is to eliminate all toxic substances.

Only spring water or distilled water was to be used, even for the enemas, though I must admit that after a while we used boiled, filtered water. Certain substances were to be avoided, including fluoridated toothpaste, underarm deodorants, and anything containing chemicals, such as insect sprays and fresh-air sprays.

Forbidden on the diet were bottled, tinned, frozen or preserved foods, in fact any food which had been de-natured by whatever process. Also forbidden were salt, commercial beverages, tea and coffee, oil, fats, nuts, mushrooms, ice-cream, (alas!) anything containing sugar, and a few other substances. Temporarily forbidden were butter, cheese, eggs, fish, meat and milk.

What could you eat? you may ask. Was there anything left? Well, yes, of course - there were salads, fruits, grains, seeds, and vegetables among some other foods, such as garlic and other herbs. Apple cider vinegar was also permitted. After an initial period of only vegan-type food, you could have buttermilk, yoghourt and cottage cheese.

Salad foods included carrots, lettuce, endive, chicory, tomatoes, cauliflower, romaine, radishes, spring onions, celery, chives and green pepper.

Fruit included apples, bananas, apricots, cherries, currants, grapes, citrus fruits, melon, peaches, pears and plums, although I found that some of these affected me, particularly plums and citrus fruit.

Peppermint tea was allowed, especially for indigestion or during a reaction period.

Sample menus were given. For breakfast you could begin with a glass of freshly squeezed juice, followed by oatmeal, cooked in water, with honey, bananas, raisins or dates, stewed fruit and/or rye bread.

For lunch you could choose any of the following:- a salad of raw vegetables, cottage cheese, a baked potato, cooked vegetables, or soup. For dessert you might have stewed or raw fruit. To drink you could have a glass of juice. The suggestions for dinner were the same as for lunch. Boiled or mashed potatoes could be substituted for baked ones.

For cancer patients liver injections were an essential part of the therapy, and also juice made from calves' liver. I tried the liver juice but it actually gave me considerable pain so I'm afraid I omitted it.

At the time I did not realise how important it was to take the liver supplements. A liver test showed an imbalance in the liver and that sulfate stores were depleted. Whether this problem started at the time I was following the detoxification programme I have no idea, but I am aware of the possibility. Through not taking the supplements to regenerate the liver I may have caused the problem. But, as I said, the liver juice gave me such pain that I discontinued it.

For diseases other than cancer four or five glasses of vegetable juice a day were recommended. The cancer patients in Dr.Gerson's care were given twelve glasses of juice a day! If you attempted this at home you would find it very hard work, not only in preparation of the juices, but in washing the juice machine between usage.

For people going to work, the suggested menu was soup, taken in a flask, fresh juice, a baked potato, and fresh mixed salad and fruit. Much fresh fruit should be taken during the day.

The utensils and cooking pots to be used should be made of stainless steel, glass, enamel, earthenware, cast iron or tin. Pressure cookers and aluminium utensils were banned. Aluminium is a poison and has been related to diseases of the nervous system and senile dementia.

On Saturday, December 30th.1989 I began the therapy in earnest.

I took no solid food, but made juice of fruit and vegetables in a juice machine lent to me by the friend who had also lent me the Gerson book. The juice machine was a centrifugal type, which although it is not the most efficient or expensive, we found served its purpose quite adequately, and were grateful for it.

The juice consisted of one cooking apple, one whole beetroot, three medium-sized carrots, about four inches of cucumber and four or five sticks of celery, as well as some green leaves, - perhaps spinach, cabbage or watercress.

The juice was varied according to what was fresh and available. The vegetables should be organic if possible, but I found these expensive and also difficult to obtain at that time, so I bought only the organic carrots, as this vegetable is especially susceptible to pollutants in the soil, such as pesticides. I found that organic carrots taste so much better than the usual ones!

The instructions for making the juice we found in a "Raw Energy" book bought from a health shop, which incidentally gives instructions as to what ingredients to use for different conditions.

As I was drinking about six glasses of juice a day, Alex helped me to make it when he was at home. I was lucky for the first ten days of the therapy, as it was his Christmas break and he was very helpful. He also helped to make the coffee for the enemas, which became easier as we progressed day by day. The theory is that the coffee opens up the bile duct and releases toxins from the bile and liver.*

After a week of following the instructions in the Gerson book I began to really feel that the toxins were leaving my body. At the same time I was taking only vegetable juices, and felt stronger and more comfortable than I had done for some time.

I began to eat solid food, - mainly raw vegetables and salads, plus the special soup made of celery, leeks, onions, potatoes and parsley. Because salt was not allowed I put garlic and other herbs into the soup.

Apart from feeling more comfortable in a physical way I was experiencing a beautiful feeling of serenity and deep peace. At the yoga and meditation group, Enid remarked, "You seem to have moved into a different space!" and I felt I had.

About three weeks after commencing the therapy, I was feeling better than I had felt for years, with more energy and stamina. In addition I did not need as much rest as I had previously been taking. This I attributed to taking the energy-giving juices. And gratifyingly other small improvements began to show themselves. A friend who sometimes gave me a massage noticed that the "knots" in my back and shoulders were not so pronounced, but added that I could "do" with a massage every day!

On the diet, I was now able to eat a greater variety of foodstuffs, even some delicious fruits such as lychees, kiwis and the occasional melon, (it was so expensive at this time of the year;) unsulphured apricots, (though later I thought that they affected me and discontinued them,) and bananas of course, which are high in potassium. I justified the extra expense of the fruit by the fact that I wasn't eating meat, eggs or cheese.

So my diet at this stage included mixed salads of raw vegetables, seeds, especially sprouted seeds, homemade vegetable soup, potatoes cooked in "jackets," some fish, herbs, ricecakes, and fruit of all kinds, although later I cut down on certain "acid" fruits. The fruits which seemed to do the least harm were sweet, ripe pears, bananas and melon, which was a special treat. This (melon) is also excellent in cleansing the digestive system.

Each day I took a variety of tablets, mainly minerals and vitamins. These included iron, Vitamin C, K Compound for potassium, (from the Arthritic Association), and lactobacillus acidopholus for the candida problem.

Although the Gerson therapy advised you to stop the drugs I was very wary of doing so, in view of my previous experience, when I had ceased all the medication and six weeks later found myself in bed with severe pain and inflammation. So this time I continued taking plaquenil which had been prescribed for me some time previously, and also voltarol as required.

Both Alex and I were having a very busy time preparing the vegetables for the juices, actually making the juice and in addition doing the normal cooking for him and Nick, our son. As well as this there were the enemas to prepare and administer every day. I would not advise anyone to embark on this therapy without a lot of thought and determination; you need a great deal of perseverance, plenty of time, and if possible a helper, as it is extremely hard work and very tiring if you are not healthy anyway. You also need to budget a certain amount of money; as well as the initial outlay for a juice machine and enema kit, you need to buy a plentiful supply of fresh vegetables, preferably organic.

The near-miraculous results of all this hard work really became apparent by the end of January. I made a list of all the self-evident improvements:-

1. The remainder of an abscess in the gum, which had been present for months, had almost disappeared.

2. The pain had disappeared from a place in the armpit where a cyst had been removed.

3. The thrush (candida) was much improved.

4. My weight had dropped from around ten stones to 8st.12lb. and moving around was much easier.

5. Some tenderness in my head, which had been bothering me for some time, had diminished.

6. Best of all, I felt stronger, fitter and more comfortable than I had felt for years.

According to Arnold Ehret, it takes between one and three years to completely cleanse the body system, but already I was feeling some positive effects!

As the toxins left my body, I began to become more conscious, more aware of what I was eating and drinking, trying to have everything as pure and uncontaminated as possible; - the freshest of vegetables, from the garden when available.

To ensure that the vegetables are in peak condition, it is important to have the shortest time possible between growing and consuming, as the nutritional value quickly diminishes, as well as the vital energy contained in the plants. I ate no processed foods and avoided additives and preservatives, as far as I knew. To drink, apart from the juices and spring water, I took herbal teas, usually peppermint.

Apart from the therapy I was having a busy time seeing friends and entertaining visitors, as well as attending my customary groups when possible, as I thought it important to keep up with my interests. These included the Environment Group of the local U.3.A., (an organisation for the over 50's,) the White Eagle Group and the ever-helpful Yoga where I met kindred spirits.

The most pain I was experiencing at this time was in the knees, and the muscles of the arms. The physiotherapy I had tried had not helped a great deal. The reason for the arm problem was probably over-use, as every day there was so much food preparation. I was so grateful for my cleaning lady who came once a week to do the basic cleaning, change the beds, and especially the ironing, as this exacerbated the arm problem. So with all the tasks, I just endeavoured to take everything steadily, without rushing.

On February 14th I recorded that the bumps on my wrists had decreased, also that the knees were feeling considerably better.

About the same time I began to take spinach juice. Raw spinach is supposed to build up the organs of the body which have been damaged. Cooked spinach does not have the same effect, in fact, according to Leslie and Susanna Kenton in their book "Raw Energy", it can actually cause disintegration of the bones.

One morning, while cleaning my room I found, among the bottles of pills, the eye drops and also mouth gel, then realised I hadn't needed to use either of these for weeks, since I had neither sore eyes nor a sore tongue!

However, I *was* anaemic. At the rheumatology department of the hospital, where I regularly attended for blood tests, weight and general check-up, the nurse phoned to ask me to attend for a stomach inspection, as my blood count was low and it was possible that I had an ulcer. The inspection would involve having a tube put down the throat into the stomach. Not a comfortable prospect!

Instinctively I felt that almost certainly there was no ulcer. I had no symptoms of one. More than likely the problem was caused by the lack of iron in my diet, combined with the effects of the enemas. Anaemia is a common occurrence with arthritis in any case. So I took a note round to the hospital to say that I was bombarding my body with iron, in the form of tablets, spinach juice, apricots, etc, etc. Also I started to take blackstrap molasses, which are excellent for iron content.

One of the reasons for the simple anaemia was probably due to the intensive use of the enemas, which remove nutritional substances in the colon before they have been properly absorbed into the body. The realisation that this was happening prompted me to reduce the number of enemas; this had two effects, one good, one disheartening!

The "good" effect was that I felt stronger and more energetic, but at the same time there was an increase in the stiffness and pain, especially in the elbows. Something I was eating was affecting me, I thought.

For some time I had suspected that *oats* were causing pain, as the stiffness was more marked after eating muesli or porridge. When I left it out of the diet I felt much better. But there were many other culprits, too.

One day in March I was in bed with pain, mentally recalling what I had eaten the previous day which might be responsible. I remembered eating a small piece of cheese in the evening. Of course that must be it!

It usually took about twenty-four hours for the effects of an allergenic substance to subside, and I would usually feel the effects for a whole day, often unable to go out of the house or even to perform my household tasks.

But if I took an enema the effects would disappear very quickly, as the toxic substance was removed from the body. The enemas, though, were also removing essential vitamins and minerals, such as iron. The effects of this often caused weakness and lack of stamina. You can't win, I thought!

By this time I had modified the Gerson diet, as I found that too much juice (vegetable and fruit), as well as being very expensive, was causing "griping" pains in the stomach, which together with diarrhoea was extremely weakening. So I cut down the amount of juice to two or three glasses a day, and felt somewhat better for it.

Apart from the juice, other drinks included herbal tea, (mainly peppermint,) and bottled spring water, as the chemicals in the tap water affected me badly, as well as tasting most unpleasant. I had noticed this only recently, probably because the cleansing of my body had made me more sensitive to the taste of chemicals. I had a filter jug and used the water from this for boiling, also for washing vegetables and fruit.

Because my skin was showing signs of dryness I increased the amount of oily fish such as herrings and mackerel, which are nutritionally excellent as well as being delicious to eat. I also took cod liver oil. I had discovered that fish oil is probably the best source of "fat" for arthritis. Through experience I knew that butter and other solid fats aggravated the condition. Later I was to learn that *all* animal fats are bad for arthritis.

It was three months since I had started the therapy. On April 5th. I recorded that I had not had a "bad" day for five days! And I was learning quite a lot about my body and the substances which affected it.

*The enema equipment we obtained from the Wholistic Research Company. (Address at end of book.) There are several types available. The instructions for use can be found in their interesting little book, "A Harmony of Science and Nature." (See Bibliography.)

A note about the enemas. When you take a plain water enema, the balance of the intestinal flora is disturbed, as the natural micro-organisms which live in the gut are washed away. Nowadays a good colonics practitioner will re-introduce the required substances back into the bowel and intestines. These bacteria, lactobacillus and lacto bio-bifidum maintain the balance of the natural micro-organisms, helping to prevent an overgrowth of candida, for instance. Live yoghourt also contains these beneficial bacteria.

CHAPTER 4.
MAKING PROGRESS

Although I was making excellent progress, I was still on drug medication. It was my avowed intention to wean myself from these until I could manage without them completely.

You may wonder why it was so important to me to be free of taking arthritis drugs.

Most drugs (if not all) have side-effects and I knew from experience how complicated this problem can become. A friend of mine who had been taking drugs for many years had developed some most unpleasant disorders; her kidneys were leaking protein and she had to have blood transfusions on a regular basis. This problem was attributed to taking Voltarol, probably the most common drug prescribed for arthritis. As for myself, taking antibiotics for various infections over the years had almost certainly precipitated the thrush (candida) which had dogged me for years.

In his book "Arthritis -The Allergy Connection," Dr.John Mansfield describes the effects of drugs on the body.

"The first-line approach to the arthritic problem, irrespective of the form of arthritis, is either aspirin or the non-steroidal anti-inflammatory drugs. Aspirin has well-known gastric side-effects taken in large dosage and all the non-steroidal anti-inflammatory drugs have a very high incidence of side-effects."

Cannot the drugs be used to heal the patient?
In Dr.Mansfield's words,

"None of these drugs eradicates arthritis or even beneficially changes its progress. There has even been a report in The Sunday Times containing evidence collected by Dr.Paul Dieppe of Bristol University that this category of drugs could lead to a prolongation of the disease process. In other words, it appears that these drugs could inhibit the natural healing processes that tend to occur in the normal situation."

Other drugs used, especially to treat rheumatoid arthritis include Cortisone, Penicillamine and Gold.

With regard to these, Dr.Mansfield says,

"These can beneficially alter the course of the disease but they are all very potent drugs with a high incidence of side-effects and occasional fatalities. These drugs are normally employed only with the more desperate patients because of the risks involved."

****

On April 12th. I attended the rheumatology department for my usual check-up. The doctor seemed quite pleased with my condition, asked me what I was eating and made a note of it. I took my courage in both hands and asked if we could reduce the plaquenil and/or the gold injections, which I was still receiving every fortnight.

The doctor asked, "Which would you prefer?"
"Plaquenil," I replied.
"You can drop it altogether," he declared.

You can imagine my delight. I was so pleased, though a little wary. Conscious that I would have to make the maximum effort to aid the healing process, I was determined to be more relaxed, to "go with the flow" in order to keep myself in balance. This was very difficult sometimes as the vibrations in the house were often not conducive to peace; the television was on nearly all the time in the evenings for one thing. So I usually went to my bedroom where it was peaceful and quiet. There I could read, meditate , practise yoga exercises or just relax.

****

On Easter Sunday, a pleasant, quiet day for me, I suddenly realised that a pain which I had experienced intermittently for years seemed to have almost disappeared, - I had not felt it for some time.

This discomfort, a tenderness in the lower right side of the abdomen, (I found out later it was in the area of the ileo-caecal valve,*) had started in 1983, about six months before the first symptoms of rheumatoid arthritis showed themselves. After visiting my G.P. in connection with this, he had referred me to a consultant.

All the usual tests were performed, including a bowel x-ray, but nothing seriously wrong was discovered. When I went for the results the consultant remarked that I was "constipated." This puzzled me as I had not had any trouble in this direction. I was "regular"!

Now I know that a state of constipation can exist even when bowel movements appear to be normal, as waste matter can accumulate somewhere along the line of the colon. In the book, "Colon Health," Dr. Norman Walker stresses that constipation is the primary cause of nearly every ailment or disturbance of the human system, affecting the health of the colon, upon which the entire health of the body depends.

Some years later, this connected in my mind with what I had read in information from the Arthritic Association, among other sources. I quote from "Rheumatic Review", September 1979:-

"Understand that the disease begins in the bowel. Incorrect diet causes: A deficiency of potassium in the blood, leading to: the muscles becoming stiff,cramped and contracted affecting the joints which are drawn closer together. Later the joints become calcified".

So what is "calcified"?
In "Rheumatism and Arthritis- the Conquest", by Charles de Coti-Marsh, the author states,

"Calcification is the collection of extraneous lime from food and waters that enter the body via the mouth and are contained in certain foods and drinks".

****

Towards the end of April I had a fall in the bedroom. I had just plugged in the telephone in order to make some calls when I caught my foot in the wire and fell headlong onto the floor, on my right side.

The sound of the crash when I fell brought Alex rushing up the stairs to see what had happened. My first thought was for my replaced hips! Had I done any damage? There was some pain in the right hip and knee, also a swelling on the hip. The soreness seemed to be localised, so it did not appear to be serious. On visiting my G.P., she confirmed that no real damage had been done, adding that I had been very lucky.

I would have to be more careful in future.

****

The knees were still an ongoing problem, especially in bed at night. I would fill a hot-water bottle and place it between the knees when I lay on my side. There are also pouches you can buy, small gel-filled "cushions", which you place into hot water, then apply to the affected area. If you prefer a cold application the pouches can be put in the fridge. For myself, the well-used bags of frozen peas have been invaluable when sitting relaxing; the same bag has been returned to the fridge and used many times! The bag may be placed on the shoulder, wrist or any other inflamed and painful area.

For a long time, I had been aware of the connection between the over-use of muscles and joints with increased pain. You might think that this is obvious, but this problem often does not show itself until afterwards. You often do not realise at the time that you are overdoing it with the gardening, or whatever activity it is. What is normal use to a healthy person may be over-use to a person with problems in the joints and muscles.

I often experienced more pain when I had been doing a lot of writing, including typewriting. This caused soreness around the right shoulder-blade, a trouble spot for several years, also in the muscles of the upper arm. Other activities which aggravated this included preparing vegetables; rubbing, e.g. cleaning saucepans; gardening (alas!) or any other activity which used the muscles to excess. The difficulty was to stop the activity before it affected me unduly. I would think to myself, "I'll just do this", or "I'll just finish that..."

From what I have written you may think I was doing nothing else apart from therapy on myself. But my life was full of other interests. There were my friends to go walks with, sometimes in the woods to see the bluebells or just for the fresh air and exercise. I was attending my usual groups; the yoga and White Eagle groups and the Environment group, which I always found interesting. Sometimes I took Peter, a disabled friend, out into Derbyshire, and we would enjoy a "pub" lunch together. Life was full of interest and activity!

****

In June, I attended the rheumatology department as usual. At each attendance at the clinic the E.S.R. (Erythrocite Sedimentation Rate) is checked, which gives an indication of the severity of the disease. A high E.S.R. (over 30 or so) suggests that the disease is quite active.

In January my E.S.R. had been forty-five, which was considered high. The following month it had dropped to forty-one, then in March it was thirty; in April twenty-six and now, on this June day, I was told that in May the marker had been twenty-five. It had dropped twenty points in four months! This was extremely encouraging.

When following the Gerson therapy, sometimes a healing crisis occurs. This phenomenon involves a feeling of nausea, with some vomiting; maybe also an attack of diarrhoea. It is actually the body's way of ridding itself of poisons and is a good sign, although it may not feel like it at the time!

When this happened to me one day, I checked in the Gerson book as I suspected it was part of the healing process. Sure enough, the symptoms were described exactly; ...vomiting, headache and sweating.

I did not feel like eating or even drinking anything, just wanting to rest in bed all day. In the evening I had some peppermint tea and a grated apple, then two Milk of Magnesia tablets before going to sleep. The next morning I felt much better.

****

As I became cleaner inside, there was a corresponding increase in the mobility and flexibility of my body. Six months after starting the therapy I recorded that I was able to cut my toe-nails on both feet! I could not remember when I was last able to do this, but it had been some time before the hip operation. This was progress indeed!

The medication I was taking at this time included gold injections, which had been reduced to one per fortnight instead of weekly; Voltarol one a day; iron, acidopholus for the candida, and potassium ("K Compound" from the Arthritic Association).

In August when I saw the rheumatologist I told him what I had done to improve my condition and also about the reduced pain in the lower right abdomen. I was convinced that when the pain had entirely disappeared through the elimination of toxins I would be well on the way to being healed.

There was a student present on this occasion and the doctor pointed out to him the swollen ligaments behind the knees, which were still giving me trouble.

Apart from the knees and the left elbow, which was also painful, there were rheumatic "knots" in my back and shoulders, which were exacerbated by certain activities such as writing, ironing, or preparing vegetables.

I found that something which helped to alleviate this was massage. A L.I.F.E. Foundation lady, Barbara, was staying with us every Monday night during this period, as she was studying an Art Therapy course in Sheffield. She was an expert masseuse, so every Monday evening she gave me a lovely, soothing massage. In between times Alex often assisted the process by massaging my back and shoulders. He always seemed to find the right spots! This gave me considerable relief and I always felt better for it the following day.

In September I noticed that some tingling in my spine, which I had felt for some time, had disappeared. By this time most days were comparatively "good", especially after taking Detox tablets or an enema the previous evening. However, I had realised by this time that too much cleansing, in the way of enemas, could be counter-productive, as nutrition is removed from the colon before it has been absorbed into the system. This was especially important when one had eaten top-grade raw food and then took an enema a few hours later. The food would be passed out before it had supplied the body with its energy-giving properties. Therefore it was better to take an enema straight after a meal, when the valuable nutrients were still in the stomach.

The reason for the enemas was of course to remove substances which caused pain, and they certainly did help to relieve discomfort and even stiffness from the body, to a considerable extent, by cleansing the system.

Another way to cleanse the system on a regular basis is by fasting.

Many people have a problem with fasting, thinking that if you miss a few meals you may starve! But fasting has a wonderful cleansing effect on the body, helping to eliminate toxins.

In his book, "The Mucousless Diet Healing System", Arnold Ehret describes in detail what happens during a fast.

The body is continually obstructed by unnatural over-pressure on the blood and to the tissues, caused by overeating. As soon as you stop eating, this pressure is relieved, the blood becomes more concentrated and the superfluous water is eliminated. The mucous and toxins in the system start to be dissolved and this waste is brought back into circulation to be eliminated.

What else happens during a fast?

A beautiful cleansing process takes place, as the little "pockets" in the colon contract and start to squeeze out any accumulated material, some of which may have been there for years, poisoning the bloodstream. According to Ehret, the pain during a fast is caused when the loosened waste and toxins go back into circulation before being eliminated by the kidneys. This process can be helped by the use of enemas and/or laxatives. This state lasts for only a day or two, and at least you know that the effects are working!

The Arthritic Association advise a fast on one day a week. The evening before a fast day, two or three Detox tablets are taken. These help to loosen the toxins and clear the colon in preparation for the fast.

On the fast day, only juices are taken, or some fresh fruit. It is preferable to take only one sort of fruit, e.g. melon or pears. Some people can take oranges, but I cannot. In the evening after a fast more Detox tablets are taken. These have the effect of clearing out waste material.

After a fast it is important to eat the right sort of food, to help to eliminate the waste matter. A vegetable soup or raw and starchless vegetables are the best, and some fresh fruit. The meal should be of a laxative nature. In the days following a fast it is usual to feel well, with renewed energy.

****

By November I was having more comfortable nights than I had experienced for years, and reasonably good days, although of course I was still taking drugs - the Voltarol and gold injections.

To my joy, I was finding greater ease in walking, so I spent a good deal of time in the park, sometimes feeding the ducks or strolling along the paths; other times walking as fast as I could, just for sheer pleasure.

I was learning to listen more to my body. Sometimes my mind and body were in conflict; my mind was telling me to do some "work", calligraphy perhaps, and I would really wish to do this, but the body would say, "You are tired, go and have a rest *now!*" I soon learned that if I did not listen to my body I would pay for it later, with pain and/or fatigue.

Since the small accident in my bedroom I was also very aware of taking care not to fall or injure myself in any way, as all the good could be undone in an instant.

****

Christmas was approaching, and one of the groups to which I belonged had arranged a Christmas lunch at a local hotel. Knowing that some of the food might affect me, I nevertheless made the decision to attend, as I would see some friends and enjoy the social occasion. I was prepared to eat just the vegetables if necessary, although the rest of the meal might be an interesting experiment!

The meal began with some tinned tomato soup, followed by "processed" turkey steak (which was extremely salty), tinned carrots, peas of a pebble-like hardness, and well-roasted potatoes. This unremarkable course was followed by an indifferent Christmas pudding, brandy sauce and coffee. I hadn't eaten such poor food for a very long time.

In the evening after returning home I made myself a salad of grated carrots, apple and celery, with water-cress, lettuce, spring-onions, raisins, bean-sprouts and almonds. It tasted wonderful!

****

On December 12th., at my usual visit to the rheumatology department I told the doctor about some tingling sensations I had been feeling, in my ear and the side of the head. This is sometimes a reaction to taking drugs. The doctor therefore made a decision to stop the gold injections. This was music to my ears! I had been on these injections for several years, and as well as the inconvenience of having to go regularly to the hospital, of more importance to me was having to rely on drugs to "help". I had thought that the injections had made very little difference, in any case.

On some days I began to feel really physically well, "on top of the world" even. I was enjoying my new-found comfort immensely. But then I would have an occasional "bad" day, which I could usually connect with eating unsuitable food. It was difficult to be "good" all the time, as it was Christmastime and there were social occasions, with all kinds of delicious tit-bits to tempt the appetite. On one occasion I ate some tomato and orange soup. which was absolutely delicious, but turned out to be absolutely lethal for me!

On New Year's Eve some friends and I held a meditation for world peace. In the evening I sat and looked at the moon and sky. It was a full moon and the sky looked magnificent, with pinky-grey clouds scudding across. I sang songs and felt wonderful.

I wondered what events the new year, 1991, would hold in store for us all.

*The ileo-caecal valve is situated near the right hip, close to the appendix. It is the "gateway" between the small intestine and the large intestine. After food has been digested, the residue passes through this valve to the large intestine, or colon. Now, the colon contains about three pounds of bacteria, many of which should not be present in the small intestine. The ileo-caecal valve ensures that the flow does not go backwards, but if it becomes weakened for any reason, then some of these harmful bacteria and waste matter can leak back into the small intestine, where it can be absorbed into the bloodstream. It then circulates round the body, causing stiffness and pain.

The valve can become weakened through disruptions to digestion, often caused by stress.

CHAPTER 5.
PEAKS AND TROUGHS

The new year, 1991, began for me by a re-dedication to service. This wishing to serve the planet gives me a strong sense of PURPOSE. It is something much bigger than my own little needs and "problems," and I knew so many people who needed help of one sort or another that sometimes I was able to fill a need, which I was glad to do. I will add that a "spin-off" from serving is that when we give, we receive... so much more than we give.

Having no definite plans, I was satisfied to flow with whatever occurred. I was learning to *trust*, *surrender* and *accept*, offering my thoughts, words and actions to the Universal Spirit. Once we do this wholeheartedly, any inner conflict or doubt about the course of action we should take seems to diminish. The decisions become easier.

The hardest part of this for me was THOUGHT, as I often caught myself out with an uncharitable thought about someone. I am still working on it! We are often unaware how much our thoughts have an influence on people and events around us and even more, of course, of the effect they have on ourselves. Watching our thoughts is so important for our personal growth.

****

As described in the previous chapter, the most pain I was having at this time was in the right shoulder and shoulder blade, made worse by preparing vegetables and other household tasks, which were part and parcel of everyday living.

In spite of the difficulties I decided to do two things. The first was to decrease the amount of the only drug I was still taking, - Voltarol, and at the same time, to compensate for this by increasing the amount of raw food and juices. I also booked for an acupuncture session.

After the first acupuncture treatment in February there was initially little noticeable difference in the amount of pain, but then, four days later I woke up feeling better, - very free and easy with hardly any pain at all! Admittedly I had taken a Voltarol tablet the previous day; I had also been exercising and dancing to music on T.V., which always causes me to feel better.

At the second session, the acupuncture practitioner mentioned that he was placing the needles in the points of tenderness and pain, which happened to follow the "colon path!" In my mind this served to reinforce the idea which had previously arisen, the concept of the connection between the colon and rheumatoid arthritis.

The acupuncture really began to take effect after this session, enabling me to abstain from the Voltarol for longer periods, - about five days on average.

In spite of the pain in shoulders and knees I was finding pleasure in performing everyday tasks and duties. Alex's nephew had arrived in May from Yugoslavia to live with us and I was enjoying preparing the food for three men and presenting it in the best way I could. So apart from seeing friends and doing occasional artwork I was considerably well-occupied in the house.

Having an extra person at home brought some changes and challenges, but I was determined to view these as opportunities, looking to see what lesson was wrapped up in each situation. And there were some lessons!

In September we had the busiest week I could remember for years. Christina, our daughter was home so there was a party organised for about twenty young people.

Some of the guests stayed for several nights, then two days later Christina's German colleague turned up in his camper van and slept in the driveway - in the van of course! So we spent an extremely eventful week, meeting some interesting people. In spite of all the activity I was not experiencing undue pain as I had followed the usual routine of fasting, diet and juices.

The most exciting event and achievement for me during this year came in September.

At the L.I.F.E. Conference in July, one of the speakers had been an extremely interesting man, a climber of international standing, who delivered a riveting talk about his life and interests.

After having experienced two near-death accidents while climbing, he had decided to spend the rest of his life in service to humanity. He had therefore devised a project, "Climb for the World", in which anyone could take part. Within twenty-four hours on a certain date, from noon Saturday to noon Sunday, volunteers would climb hills and mountains to raise money for international projects. This was done by each volunteer being given a sponsor sheet to be filled in by friends and relatives.

The projects seemed immensely worthwhile. One was to access water for villages in India; another was to help protect the rainforests, a project close to my heart. I dearly wanted to take part in this.

Quite near to where we live are the beautiful hills of Derbyshire, some of which were included in the list of suggested "mountains" to walk or climb up.

So, on September 21st., 1991, four friends, with a baby carried in a back-pack, and myself, set off to climb up one of these hills, a feat which I hadn't tackled since the start of the arthritis. We chose for the venture a lowish plateau called Stanage Edge, the easiest way up being a sloping footpath followed by a scramble up some gritstone rocks.

The weather was sunny but a strong wind was blowing. My friend Eirlys, firmly holding one end of one of my husband's golf clubs, and I, holding tightly to the other, slowly and carefully made our way along the heather-skirted footpath. When we reached the steep rocky edge of the plateau I released my hold on the club as it was necessary to use both hands to steady myself as I gingerly picked my way up the rocks.

As we approached the top, my feelings were indescribable. On the plateau the almost gale-force wind accelerated my sense of exhilaration and elation. How wonderful it was to be up there! I could not remember when I last experienced such a feeling of buoyancy and well-being.

We could not stand too near the edge of the plateau because of the dangerous wind, although we were able to see the amazingly beautiful view of Hope Valley, the purple heather-covered hills and green fields, home to Derbyshire sheep.

Nearby, in a tent especially erected for the occasion, "World Passports" were stamped, then we wrote peace messages to the world. I had prepared my message, which said, "Peace begins with the individual and can only be found by releasing any resentment or bitterness in the heart. Only by this can we live together as brothers and sisters, children of this beautiful planet, which we should cherish and care for as the precious inheritance that it is."

What a wonderful day I had had! The thought arose that even a year previously I would not have been able to take part in this tremendous event, and I was so grateful to my friends for helping and sharing it with me.

The following day I was especially delighted to discover that my body had not suffered unduly from the exercise, in fact I felt quite well.

****

The autumn was a busy time for us, as among other things we were having a patio made, by a friend, John. This involved planning and designing it ourselves and it was a source of interest to see how it was evolving day by day. John is a good worker and I was kept busy making endless cups of tea to keep him going!

As well as the usual groups I attended I was going to a "lunch club" one day a week, to talk to a deaf-blind man, Reg, in finger language. He was a dear, a model of patience and serenity which many sighted people would envy.

Because of all my activities I once more found myself performing tasks at a slightly faster rate than was natural to me, and so becoming "tensed up". So in the evening I would relax in a warm bath, then rest in bed with an absorbing book.

About this time I began to feel really comfortable inside, more comfortable than I had been for years. Was this the result of the internal cleansing?

However I was still "taking the tablets", and it was my dearest wish to be able to improve to the point that I did not need them any longer.

****

I celebrated New Year, 1992, by giving thanks to the Universe for the help I had received up to that moment in time, then made some affirmations and dedications.

By surrendering to a Higher Power I felt directed, - decisions were made by themselves, and in spite of challenges and difficulties because of my condition I strongly felt the presence of an ongoing, unseen daily help. I felt suffused by a great sense of love and knew that it surrounded me. I prayed for continued help in my progress and development; to conquer my *self*; to release myself from pain of any kind, fear, desires, tension or anything which would hinder the healing process. I also prayed for help to be positive in my thoughts, words and actions. From experience I had found that as soon as any negativity crept into my thinking, especially with regard to criticism or judgment, the feelings of peace and power went out "through the window."

The repetition of certain words or phrases impinges them into our consciousness until they become part of our thinking process. It is amazing what a difference this practice can make to your life. Words like *Positivity, Power, Peace* and *Joy* when regularly repeated can fill you with a wonderful sense of mastery over yourself, a feeling of being able to accomplish anything you wish to do. This practice seems to empower you with a tremendous feeling of calmness, peace and "centredness" with which to begin the day; this attitude then affects other people with whom you come into contact, then is spread to others and so on, like ripples on a lake.

****

Early in the year I was referred to the Physiotherapy Department at the hospital for treatment on my hands, as the fingers are curved inwards, especially the little fingers of both hands. The treatment involved immersing the hands in warm paraffin wax, holding them up to dry then peeling the wax off like gloves, rolling it into a ball and manipulating it to exercise the hands, along with other hand and finger exercises. The wax has a lovely effect on the skin, leaving it silky and smooth.

I was supposed to do these therapeutic exercises each day. Although I did them when I remembered, usually when watching T.V., nevertheless I could not find enough time to do them as often as I would have liked, or should have done.

****

During January I had succumbed to a virus infection. This manifested as a sort of 'flu which caused dizziness, fatigue, nausea and headache, and lasted for the best part of a week, but kept returning intermittently for months, right into the following year in fact. The doctor called it "labyrinthitis," an infection of the middle ear. Whatever it was it was most unpleasant, and may have been one of the factors to cause a deterioration in my progress during the months following the first attack.

Writing, painting, gardening and other activities were causing me considerable pain and I reluctantly increased the dosage of Voltarol to one per day. I took Detox tablets and fasted one day a week to help the problem - this worked for a couple of days each time but then I would be back to "square one." Furthermore, in April I started to experience tangible pain in the right ear and right side of the head as well as in the usual places. As if this weren't enough my joints felt very stiff at night and in the mornings. By June the legs and knees were so stiff and painful that I could hardly climb the stairs to go to bed. What had gone wrong? What was causing all these problems? I asked myself.

I was aware that one of my greatest problems was candidiasis, or "Candida," as it is commonly called. To combat it, I took "live" yoghourt and acidophilus capsules every day. But what I did not know was what happens when the fungus gets "out of hand." (For more details of this, please see Appendix 1 - "Candida".)

At this time I was still eating nuts, cottage cheese, ice-cream occasionally (my favourite!), dried fruit such as dates, raisins and sultanas, an occasional egg, and a variety of fruits including apples and pears. These foods are all "banned" on a Candida diet, but in between occasional attacks of thrush and cystitis I didn't realise that the problem was so serious.

****

So the time went by; my condition fluctuated; sometimes there were comparatively "good" periods, but more frequently there were bouts of severe pain which caused me to reach for the Voltarol tablets.

It took a couple of months to recover sufficiently for me to risk reducing the Voltarol once more. But by September I had made some improvement and was managing to last for longer periods between taking the drug, - four and-a-half days, ...six days...then - a whole week! This was a milestone indeed, and extremely rewarding. It was only necessary to take the tablets if the soreness and stiffness became really uncomfortable, or if I needed to feel really well for a special occasion or day out.

I was still fruit-fasting and detoxifying once a week and now, most of the time, was beginning to feel much better internally, as the process of cleansing took place. However I really wanted to discover more about the reason for the pain and stiffness in the joints and muscles, which almost always occurred after eating certain particular foods to which I seemed to be allergic, or intolerant. And I still had to rely on the Voltarol to enable me to cope during these difficult periods.

CHAPTER 6.
TESTING FOR FOOD
ALLERGIES

For a number of years I had been aware that after eating certain foods there was increased pain and stiffness, which sometimes appeared within a short time, but often did not manifest until the following day. It did not occur to me, however, to look upon these as "allergic" reactions, as I thought of allergies in connection with such disorders as hay-fever, eczema or asthma.

However, towards the end of 1992 I ordered a book which sounded as though it might be interesting:- "Arthritis,the Allergy Connection," by Dr.John Mansfield.

(This book has been re-published as "Arthritis - Allergy, Nutrition and the Environment.") With increasing excitement and fascination I devoured the pages, as their contents yielded information which seemed to resonate with something deep inside myself; without any doubt I recognised the unmistakeable truth of it. The information given on all aspects of allergic reactions, with the research done, was extremely impressive.

Some of the research dates from many years ago, when certain doctors discovered that if a person suffers from a food allergy, and then the food was excluded from the diet altogether, there was a dramatic response in almost all cases. If the food was re-introduced after five days, the reaction returned very quickly, often within four or five hours.

Dr.Mansfield describes a "masked" allergy, where a person has withdrawn symptoms of pain after excluding the allergenic food - headaches and fatigue, before a slow improvement takes place. On the sixth day he is better.

Apart from food allergies, we can become allergic to other substances. The second greatest allergy problem is caused by *chemicals*. These can be inhaled, or are present in the food.

The chemicals in food include pesticides and insecticide sprays on fruit, which permeate the whole of the fruit, not just the skin, so it is best to buy organically grown ones if possible. The most commonly sprayed vegetables include the leafy ones:- spinach, cauliflower and broccoli, and lettuce.

Common additives include:- hydrocarbons, which contain animal fat through their feed; ethylene gas used to ripen bananas; "waxed" cucumbers, oranges, apples and peppers; chlorine in tap water, which may also contain insecticide spray; food colorants often found in ice-cream, confectionery, soft drinks, butter, margarine and many other foods. It is always advisable to read the small print before purchasing these items.

The most commonly *inhaled* allergen in rheumatoid arthritis is household gas. Other ones include sponge rubber in cushions and mattresses, and cigarette smoke, which may induce headache, nausea and fatigue.

Some inhaled allergens are present in the air we breathe. These incude pollen, house-dust, dust mites, furs, moulds, feathers and so on. It is well-known that these can cause asthma, rhinitis and hay-fever, but recently it was discovered that arthritis can be influenced by such factors.

I was eager to discover exactly which foods were affecting me, although of course certain ones had made themselves evident. So on November 30th. I began to follow Dr.Mansfield's programme.

The diet consists of a handful of foods which you normally eat only rarely, so they are unlikely to affect you. These include pears, avocados, swedes, sweet potatoes, peaches, celery, marrow, courgettes and carrots, and some fish. If you normally eat any of these more than twice a week they should be omitted. For me this meant leaving out the carrots and celery as I ate them frequently. Vegetable oil may be used, either sunflower or safflower, whichever you use less often. The only water to be drunk is bottled spring water. For seasoning, sea-salt is allowed. These are the only foods you can eat on stage one.

Apart from foodstuffs, care has to be exercised with other substances. Teeth should be cleaned with a solution of bicarbonate of soda, rather than toothpaste. The gum on stamps is made of corn starch, so these should not be licked. Of course, smoking is not allowed.

Perhaps the greatest potential problem on starting the Elimination Diet is that any drugs you are taking have to be discontinued. The reason for this is that anti-arthritic tablets almost always contain foodstuffs to which you may be allergic, such as cornflour or milk. A small amount would not normally matter, but in the first stages of an elimination diet consuming an allergenic food can have a profound effect.

Following the Elimination diet

On the first morning a large dose of Epsom Salts is taken, to clear the system of preceding food.

So having taken this, my breakfast consisted of stewed pears (without any sweetening), then nothing else apart from spring water until 5.30 p.m., when I made some juice from sweet potatoes. For dinner I cooked a fillet of cod, accompanied by parsnip and sweet potato. It tasted delicious!

On the first day there was some discomfort and general tiredness, which fluctuated during the following days; some were better than others. I followed the diet religiously, sometimes mashing the vegetables, or making juice with them, to vary it a bit.

By the seventh day I was feeling considerably better, with very little pain, although I had not taken a Voltarol for eleven days. In the evening I was to test my first food – broccoli. It tasted good, and there was no adverse reaction.

The next day was "chicken day" - I decided to have some for breakfast! About an hour later, I was out shopping when the pain and stiffness started. During the day the reaction became worse, affecting joints and muscles - right shoulder blade, left ankle, knees and other places too numerous to mention. So it seemed I was allergic to chicken. Some time later it was found that free-range chickens did not affect me in the same way. So I supposed that it was probably some substance that was <u>in</u> the chicken which was the culprit, maybe it had been injected with hormones, a common practice.

To combat a reaction, Dr.Mansfield recommends taking a dose of sodium bicarbonate mixed with potassium bicarbonate. The bicarbonate of potassium may be difficult to obtain but can be ordered from a good chemist. The quantities are two teaspoonfuls bicarbonate of soda to one teaspoonful of potassium bicarbonate. This helps to clear a reaction, and I have found it invaluable, especially when on holiday, or after visiting a restaurant where you have no control over what is put into your food, in spite of choosing carefully from the menu.

The mixture does two things:-

1) It gives you a bowel movement which helps to eliminate the allergenic food.
2) Food allergies increase the acidity in the body, which causes many of the symptoms. This alkali mixture helps to correct the acid/alkali balance in the body.

It is stressed that you should not continue testing until the reaction has cleared. A further dose of the remedy may be taken four to six hours after the initial one.

After the chicken reaction I took the prescribed dose and must admit it tasted pretty unpleasant, although I am used to it now.

In the evening the reaction started to clear and by about 3 a.m. the next morning I was feeling very much better, this was about seventeen hours after eating the chicken.

For several days I continued testing various foods with no ill-effects, until Day Eleven. This was tap water day.

I had not drunk tap water for some considerable time, as we use a filter jug which filters out most of the minerals and chemicals. For cold drinks I take bottled spring water. So it was no surprise when, about one hour after drinking the tap water the familiar pain and stiffness began. The reaction was not as severe as the chicken one had been; nevertheless I took a dose of the "bicarbs." mixture.

Over the following weeks I continued testing according to the programme. It was a relief to find that nothing affected me as severely as had the chicken and tap water, however I made some interesting discoveries.

One morning the usual reaction discomfort made itself evident. I could not think what had caused this, as all the foods taken on the previous day had been "safe," I thought. Then I remembered that I had eaten quite a lot of nuts

- almonds. Looking at a chart of acid-forming foods I found that the almonds were almost certainly the culprit, as nuts are indeed acid-forming.

Brussels sprouts are also acid-forming so I eat them only occasionally.

Another discovery was that I felt much more comfortable after eating rice. Beans - butter beans for example - had the same effect.

Acid fruits such as oranges caused a slight reaction, with a stronger one to lemons. I have since discovered that I am intolerant to plums and peaches, among other fruits. This was rather disappointing as I love fruit.

Sugar also caused a reaction and I found that anything sweet brought back the candida symptoms, so I know that sugar is more-or-less "out" for me. Some symptoms of candida often occurred after eating or drinking *anything* sweet, even if there was no "sugar" in it; this is because many fruits and vegetables contain a natural sugar, "fructose." So even sweet fruit has to be limited, as well as "acid" fruit, which could cause some considerable pain.

Some foods which caused slight reactions included eggs, cream and butter and to my dismay I experienced a strong reaction to cheese - the hard variety. Cottage cheese was more acceptable. I had always enjoyed cheese so there was no denying my disappointment. I have since found that goat's cheese does not affect me so severely.

To be honest, during all the time I was testing for food allergies there was some stiffness and pain which varied in severity. Usually it was no more than a slight discomfort, which became worse towards the evenings. Much of this, I suppose was caused by physical stress on the body, as when I am lucky enough to have a restful day there is usually very little pain on the one following.

Another reason for the continual discomfort I attributed to the discontinuation of the Voltarol, a necessary requirement for the testing. It was also possible that other allergies, apart from food, might be implicated.

Because of the stiffness in the knees and legs, on Christmas Eve I weakened and decided to take one Voltarol tablet, as we were going to be very busy on Christmas Day cooking for and entertaining family visitors; I needed to be as mobile as possible. Although I did not eat the delicious-looking turkey (I had not yet "tested" it), I enjoyed my vegetarian Christmas dinner, and we spent a happy day together.

The next day I did in fact eat some turkey and was none the worse for it! My arms were the only sufferers from Christmas, through all the food preparation.

After Christmas I tested some grains. Wheat and corn seemed to be acceptable but when I tested muesli I experienced a strong reaction. Then I recalled that I always seemed to feel worse after eating *oats*.

Another ingredient in the muesli was fruit peel, which always affected me. I always had to "vet" fruit cake very carefully!

From the results of the food testing, my dietary requirements became much clearer. Basically, this is what I had to do:-

1) Cut down dairy produce to the absolute minimum, omitting cheese altogether, except cottage cheese.
2) Leave out sugar and glucose, also reduce other sweet substances, e.g. honey.
3) Omit tap water unless I could be sure that no chemicals were added.

4) Eat more rice, raw vegetables, salads, seeds, especially sprouting seeds, and certain fruits, with preference for organic produce as the chemicals in sprays and additives affected me.

5) Omit other specific foods to which I had shown an intolerance. These included lemons, vegetable stock cubes, camomile tea, vinegar and sea-food.

6) Avoid foods containing colorings, preservatives and other chemicals, as far as I was able to ascertain.

7) Use vegetable oils for cooking, rather than solid fats.

8) For protein, apart from nuts and seeds I could eat fish, especially oily fish such as herrings, salmon or mackerel. Tinned fish was also acceptable.

With reference to raw vegetables it is now well-known that they contain vital energy, the essence of vitality derived from the sun's energy. This vital substance cannot be analysed, nevertheless it exists as a wonderful, natural source of power for us to draw upon and utilise. Raw vegetables provide a wealth of nutrition which is an invaluable healing aid to the body, keeping it in the best possible condition. In their book "Raw Energy," Leslie and Susannah Kenton recommend a diet of 75% raw food plus some wholesome cooked food. Each meal should begin with some raw food, -vegetables or fruit.

(See Chapter 11 -Diet and Vitamins.)

There are other methods of testing for allergies apart from the elimination diet, although this probably provides the most proof, if eliminating a certain food leads to a reduction in symptoms, and reintroducing it causes the problems to reoccur.

Other methods of testing for allergies include:-

1) Cytotoxic testing.

This is done by means of a simple blood test. One common reaction occurs when there is a substantial production of antibodies which respond to an antigen (allergic substance) in the blood. These antibodies (mainly IgG) appear in a long-term sensitivity or intolerance.

Cytotoxic testing is available at York Nutritional Laboratory. The blood sample can be sent by post.

2) Automated Cytotoxic Testing.

This works on a similar principle to the above, but involves an automatic haemotology unit, and the changes are analysed by computer. Since it is automated in theory it should be more reproducible (consistent).

It is available from The individual Diet Company.

3) ELISA IgG Food Sensitivity Tests.

ELISA stands for Enzyme Linked Immuno Sorbent Assay. This method claims to be the most reliable and reproducible. The disadvantage is that it is expensive.

ELISA is available from Higher Nature.

Other tests, e.g. the Intra-dermal test and the RAST test are limited in that they show some food allergies, (IgE based reactions) but many will not be identified.

Addresses can be found at the end of the book.

CHAPTER 7.
TRIALS AND TRIBULATIONS.

In addition to confirming much of what I already knew, the allergy testing provided me with new information on which to work, to aid my progress in the self-healing therapy into which I had launched myself.

In spite of putting this knowledge into practice the pain and stiffness was still "dogging" me, and fatigue was a constant companion. I always seemed to feel tired, even on waking in the morning. The juice made on the machine helped somewhat but actually feeling energetic was a rare luxury.

Part of the reason for this was the innumerable necessary household tasks to perform each day. As I tried to accomplish these as quickly as possible, in order to make time for more interesting things, I would become tense and therefore tired. So I had to rest. It was a Catch 22 situation! I found, however, that when I *gave* myself more time to do things properly, without rushing, e.g. sitting comfortably to prepare vegetables while listening to relaxing music, I felt much less stressed and the fatigue decreased. And I still had some free time in the end!

Usually, when experiencing pain in the joints and muscles, I could trace it back to something eaten the previous day. A typical example happened in March '93. The muscles were aching and "heavy", followed by a day of severe pain. The previous day a friend and I had visited a cafe and I had eaten two tiny scones with butter and jam, and some delicious ice-cream. Was it worth it? I wondered. Even these seemingly innocuous foodstuffs were sufficient to cause trouble.

When I made a cake for family or visitors, at one time I would have been able to give myself a little treat by clearing out the mixing bowl as I enjoyed the taste of the mixture, but now...I was not able to eat even the smallest amount!

When I felt well it was usually because I had taken one of the following:- a Voltarol tablet, Detox tablets, an enema, or Dr. Mansfield's "remedy". (See Chapter 6 -Testing for Allergies.) The only way to be as well as possible on a particular day, it seemed, was to take a Voltarol tablet the previous evening.

During the spring of 1993 I made more effort to keep to the strict diet regime. After a week or two this started to pay off! As the problems began to diminish, so did my need for the constant use of the Voltarol. I only took one when it was absolutely necessary, and these times became more widely spaced, so that during the summer I was managing to cope for at least a week without using it. By September I was managing a fortnight without the Voltarol prop and in November my diary records that five whole weeks had passed without my having to resort to the drug! I began to feel hopeful that at some point in the not-too-distant future it would be possible to give it up altogether.

About this time, one morning while doing the exercises to the tape I discovered that I was able to touch my right shoulder with my right hand - the first time for years!

I was making headway, slowly but surely.

It was clear that the improvement was always more marked in the summer than the winter. I don't think this was altogether connected with the weather.

On reflection I think that one reason for my progress in the summer is that there was plenty of fresh green produce in the garden, so when making juice, all I had to do was to go outside and pick some green leaves - maybe broccoli, lettuce, rocket or even dandelion and nettles! These are full of vitamins and minerals to give energy and have played an enormous part in my progress.

Another reason, I am sure, is that I spend more time outside in the summer, breathing in the fresh air, which is so important for oxygenising the body. Also sunshine has a beneficicial effect on the immune system.

However, with a disease like rheumatoid arthritis you can never be sure of *anything* in the progress department - you never know what is going to happen next. You have to learn to accept set-backs and discouragements, if you can, with equanimity and a philosophical attitude. What else can you do?

Two setbacks for me came early in the following year, 1994.

The whole family were all sitting at the dining table enjoying lunch, including our daughter Tina who was paying us a visit. I was quite comfortable, with my legs bent under the chair. But after the meal, when I tried to rise from the table I found it impossible to move; the knee was agonising and would not move in any direction. I sat there for a while wondering if I would be there for ever...! Then Nick fetched some ice which we placed on the offending knee. After a while he helped me to stand up, we heard an almighty Crack!...and I could move it. But it was so stiff I could hardly climb up the stairs. A warm bath and massage helped, but it was several days before it began to feel more normal.

Maybe the reason for this little episode was that I had been sitting in a fixed position for too long; also I had been drinking some red wine with my meal. Previously on that day I had eaten grapes and some melon, so maybe there was too much acid in the body....? Who knows?

The knee problem recurred more recently and this time with a vengeance, leading me to seek the help of a chiropractor.

One morning in the autumn I was sitting writing at the computer, my legs bent under the chair, unconscious of my position...(I must be a slow learner!) When I was ready for a break I tried to stand...and could not straighten the leg... the knee was locked. After managing to hop around the table to try to reach the phone/ go to the loo/ have a drink, I felt so faint with pain and nausea that I lay on the floor, face down. After a few moments the realisation hit me that if I was lying down, the leg must be straight! It had righted itself, but felt uncomfortably sore and stiff, so after attending to my needs I lay down for a rest.

The following day I spent a pleasant time with a friend in Derbyshire, and was pretty tired by bedtime, so climbed into bed in anticipation of a good night's sleep. I like to snuggle down with the bedclothes close round my body, so I lifted them with my knee, then ... oh no! The knee had locked again.

I tried everything I could think of to make it go straight, but this time, to my dismay, it seemed to be absolutely determined to stay in the bent position. Eventually I fell asleep out of sheer exhaustion, hoping it would right itself by morning.

Next day brought no relief so I rang the doctor from the bedside telephone, and requested a visit. When my pleasant lady doctor arrived she examined the knee, then decided not to touch it for fear of further complications, so we arranged for me to telephone the consultant who had performed the hip operation. When I phoned for an appointment the secretary explained that because the consultant was on a visit to London there was a waiting list of two and a half weeks, unless there was a cancellation. I didn't relish the prospect of being confined to my room for all that time, unable to walk, so in the meantime the G.P. was going to try to obtain an appointment for me at the Rheumatology Department of the hospital.

But when I spoke to friends on the phone, some of them recommended something I had heard about, but never experienced - chiropractic treatment. Several people described how successfully *they* had been treated by this method. So I phoned a chiropractic clinic and made an appointment for the next day, Wednesday.

At 5.15 p.m. the next day Alex wheeled me into the clinic in "my" old borrowed wheelchair. Incidentally I had often thought of returning this to the hospital where we had borrowed it, at the time before the hip operation, but something had always stopped me...now it had been useful on the five days I had been unable to walk, for use in transit between the bedroom and bathroom!

At the clinic there was a form to fill in with my personal details and health history. Then, after changing into a robe, I was wheeled into the treatment room.

The chiropractor was a pleasant young man who, after introducing himself, asked me some questions. How long had I had the rheumatoid arthritis? Which parts were affected? Had the knee "locked" before? and so on.

Normally an X-ray is taken, but in view of the fact that I was seeing the consultant next day (there had been a cancellation so my appointment had been brought forward), and he would also probably take X-rays, the chiropractor decided to forego it.

I was asked to lie on the couch while the chiropractor examined the knee and compared it with the other one. Then he started the treatment - jerking, manipulating, pulling the leg and so on, always being aware of the replaced hips. And, as he worked, the leg started to straighten. I was so delighted I began to laugh. Of course there was some pain but the relief seemed to bubble up in me, coming out as laughter! The practitioner kept saying, "I'll just do this", or "I'll just do that", until the leg was more-or-less straight. It still felt sore, of course, but I walked out of the clinic pushing the chair I had arrived in!

Naturally I felt a little trepidation as to whether the knee would "lock" again, so I took great care of it. Most mornings I exercised it in a warm bath, followed by a massage with special oil containing lavender. I had to treat the other knee as well as the strain of walking differently was causing some problems.

Each day showed an encouraging improvement. This was enhanced by further treatment at the clinic, and soon the knee began to feel comfortable once more, as the pain decreased. I felt that the treatment fee had been money well spent.

As well as massaging the knees manually, I had the help of a massage machine which my daughter had once given me; it is like a hand-held hair dryer. I would sit on the bed with the machine propped up against the knees, and while it was "doing its stuff" I massaged my hands, wrists and elbows at the same time. This routine was followed for many weeks with excellent results.

After the first time the knee locked, (as if that wasn't enough!) another incident happened in March, the evening before my birthday. I was frying chips in the kitchen for one of the "boys" when the pan slid off and uptilted, empty-ing all its contents of boiling oil onto my feet. Mirko, my husband's nephew who lives with us, immediately brought a bowl of cold water and I kept the feet immersed in this for about four hours, more or less. On going to bed the pain was agonising! In spite of taking two paracetamol tablets and some Rescue Remedy, it was some time before I was able to fall asleep. In fact sleep only came when I made myself relax "into the pain".

A couple of days later I decided to visit my G.P. as the blisters were bursting and there could be a risk of infection. This is always a problem when you have had joint replace-ment as infection can settle in that area. Even if you have a tooth removed you are advised to take antibiotics, which really "goes against the grain" with me as I have a history of episodes of thrush (candida), which is always exacerbated by taking antibiotics, depending on which ones they are. So I am very wary of taking them.

After the doctor prescribed the antibiotics a nurse came regularly to dress the feet, until the day came when it was possible for me to drive down to the surgery. On one occa-sion the nurse remarked that it was a "good job" I was taking the antibiotics as the feet were so "messy!" The wound on the right ankle was quite deep, and altogether it took several months before my feet were looking "themselves" again.

The months following this occurrence saw me at a standstill with regard to making progress. The shoulders, arm muscles, elbows, hands and wrists were all as bad as ever, but the worst pain of all was in the knees. In addition to that I had some symptoms of candida, possibly exacer-bated by the antibiotics I had taken earlier in the year.

What I did not realise was that this last problem, the candida, might be a sort of pointer as to why I was not making headway with the therapy.

If you have ever climbed a mountain, and on approaching what you thought was the summit, only to discover that there were more peaks ahead, you will understand my feelings...

CHAPTER 8.
KINESIOLOGY

In August, 1994 my long search for a "cure" for rheumatoid arthritis led me to a Kinesiologist, Ralph Pike.

Ralph has been actively involved with natural health for over eight years and owns a health shop in Sheffield. He has a diploma in Professional Kinesiology, the course of which included the study of Nutrition, Clinical Medicine, Anatomy and Physiology, Counselling Skills, Polarity, Reflex Analysis and the Vital Force/Chakra Balance, as well as the basic Balanced Health Kinesiology, together with advanced techniques.

So what exactly is Kinesiology?

In Ralph's own words, "Kinesiology is a relatively new discipline that has been in development since 1965. Based on natural healing therapies such as acupuncture,...Kinesiology draws together many tools in order to investigate the way our bodies function.

"Having determined where imbalances may lie, Kinesiology then offers gentle and non-invasive methods of correction, taking into account all aspects of the person being treated."

How is it done?

"The whole basis of Kinesiology relies on the accurate assessment of particular muscles and the way they function.

Virtually all of the muscle tests performed are standard physiotherapy techniques, although the emphasis is somewhat different.

"Having placed either the arm or the leg in an exact position, the Kinesiologist will then demonstrate the range of motion in which the limb will be moved. Basically, there will be a gentle and gradual 'push' from the tester in order to move the limb in that particular direction. The role of yourself is to resist this force to the limit of comfort.

I push one way - you push the exact opposite way."

If the resistance to pressure is difficult or painful, the limb is relaxed and allowed to move. The process is merely an assessment of one's ability to resist a gentle pressure with ease.

When particular muscles test "weak", this can indicate where imbalances in the body lie. Sometimes foodstuffs and other substances, such as herbal remedies, are placed on the body for testing. This procedure can alter muscle function whereby a previously "strong" muscle becomes "weak", or vice versa.

The treatment might begin immediately upon the Kinesiologist finding some imbalances in the body. It would usually consist of lightly touching parts of the body (normally on the head), or gently massaging specific points situated around the body

Following treatment, it is not unusual for dietary changes to be suggested, together with vitamin, mineral or other therapy if indicated. The regime may be simple and inexpensive, or rather complex and expensive, but there is no obligation to do either. You may simply be given some massage homework to do for a few days or weeks!

How can you be tested if you are disabled or very young?

I quote, "This can be overcome with surrogate testing, whereby another person is tested on behalf of the actual patient whilst maintaining skin (and therefore electromagnetic) contact with the patient. In this instance, the surrogate tests as the patient would - NOT as they themselves would. Corrections are applied to the patient."

A comprehensive health questionnaire is given to the patient to fill in, prior to attendance.

The first session normally lasts about an hour and a half; the subsequent sessions about 30 minutes to an hour. The number of sessions needed is of course subjective, but some idea may be gained at the first meeting, and passed on to the patient.

Kinesiology may be used to treat numerous conditions, including Food Allergies, Stress and Tension, Anaemia, Constipation, Sciatica, Back and Neck Ache, Headaches, Insomnia, Depression, M.E., Weight Problems, Tennis Elbow and many other disorders.

The techniques Ralph uses are of course based on Kinesiology, used in conjunction with other complementary disciplines. However, a variety of remedies are used. As well as vitamins, herbs, minerals, and the vital nutrition therapy, homoeopathy is used when appropriate. Other remedies might include the use of Essential oils, Bach flower remedies, Gem remedies and Chakra balancing.

Ralph firmly believes that your individual body has the knowledge within itself to attain good health. His work is to access that information so that a natural increase in health and vitality can be achieved.

The catalyst which led me to seek his help had been put into motion several months previously.

On a visit to a workshop at Kirkby Fleetham Hall, North Yorkshire, in June, 1994, I had learned from two separate sources that candida, which had dogged me for years, was now regarded as completely curable. If I had been on the "right" grapevine I would have known this several years previously.

One source of this information was a magazine article which described some treatment developed and used in a German clinic, which involved the use of drugs. Being by nature averse to using drugs if at all possible this didn't sound too attractive to me and I determined to find an alternative way of combating the problem.

Trying to follow up the other source of information proved unsuccessful, but if necessary I would follow this up again.

So, in Sheffield, I went to the local herbalist's shop, which happened to be owned by Ralph, and asked what treatment they presently advised for candida.

Caroline, the assistant, who incidentally had been one of my pupils in years gone by, told me that Ralph was able to treat candida successfully, but it was necessary for me to see him in order to discover the best treatment for my individual case. So I made an appointment.

As I was a regular customer in the shop, I had already met Ralph and had actually seen a demonstration of Kinesiology in which he had taken part. I knew him as a personable, likeable, family man with a good deal of knowledge of complementary therapies and holistic medicine. I also knew his wife, Sandra, who leads an extremely busy life, combining looking after Ralph and their three small children with helping in the shop, all done with supreme calmness and unruffled good humour.

At the first session we began with an interview, where all kinds of questions were asked. Why was I there?

I mentioned several reasons and was asked to identify the most important one. I could not decide between the candida and the arthritis, but plumped for candida as, thinking it might be a crucial factor in the arthritis, would have to be treated first. Ralph asked me what were the symptoms? How long had I had it? When did the arthritis start? What things made it a) better, b) worse?

The interview lasted for about half an hour, then I was asked to lie on the treatment couch. I asked for a pillow to place under the knees. Then Ralph asked me to bend and straighten my right arm while he did a test with a magnet.

Explaining that this test worked with the anterior deltoid muscle, and noting that since I was not able to straighten the arm properly, thus causing other muscles to be brought into play, he would be unable to obtain a true "reading." Although he could use a leg rather than an arm, the testing was rather lengthy and would not be "user friendly" to me, having joint pains in the knees particularly. So Ralph asked me if I would mind if we used a surrogate, Sandra, who was available as the sessions were held in their house. I agreed to this.

Sandra lay on the couch while I sat on the opposite side of the couch from where Ralph stood. I was asked to place my hand on the skin of her left arm. Then the testing began.

The tests included rheumatoid arthritis (positive); candida (positive and a considerable amount); candida toxins (positive); the medications I was presently taking.

Ralph discovered by testing that the greatest problem at that time was the toxins in my body, so this would have to be treated first.

As he tested the medications, if one was all right Ralph left the container on Sandra's body, so that he could ascertain if others were compatible or contra-indicated, even if they were all right on their own.

Some of my tablets contained sugar, or were sugar-coated, such as the iron (Ferrous Gluconate) tablets bought at the chemist's, also the echinacea, which I take to help boost the immune system. Another brand of echinacea without sugar coating was O.K. I was tested for lactose and gluten which were both positive, in other words they would affect me. Ralph also tested me for protozoa and worms, both of which are common problems, as these parasites are frequently present in the gut. I was also tested to find which places in the body were affected by the candida. Then I was tested for some foodstuffs.

One of my tablets was "garlic" and this was found to affect me. So Ralph then tested me for both garlic and onions; these were both pronounced positive, much to my disappointment, as I used them regularly in cooking, and knew the beneficial health effects of garlic in particular.

I told him that I thought something in the vegetable juice that I made was suspect, so he tested me for the ingredients. Carrot, celery and cucumber were O.K., also cabbage and lettuce. The only other regular ingredient was raw beetroot, but there was none to hand at that moment. I had suspected beetroot because, in spite of it giving me energy, it tasted sweet and therefore contained natural sugar, which having the same effect as refined sugar, should be take with caution if you have a candida problem.

Another test was performed to see if I *wanted* to get well. It was a relief to find that I did! This isn't as obvious as it sounds, because some people really do not wish to be better; they may have all sorts of veiled and/or complicated reasons for this, some of which they may not even realise themselves.

Ralph then tested his own remedies to find ones suitable for me to take for the disorders present in my body. When an appropriate one was found, there were tests for strength and dosage. Sandra was extremely patient and good-natured; indeed she proved to be exactly the same on subsequent visits.

The whole session lasted more than two hours, and had been fascinating. I left with a sheet of information on candida and an advice sheet recommending which foods and medication to take, and which to avoid.

The main medications to take were some specialised herbal complexes for the protozoa, and also for the candida toxins. Optional ones included iron, Quercetin (for the immune system), my usual K Compound (potassium), and Acidopholus, for the candida.

Foods to avoid included potatoes, tomatoes, peppers, aubergines, milk, onions, garlic, lactose and gluten, the latter being found in wheat, oats, rye and barley, but not in bran, so I would be able to take oat bran. Tobacco belongs to the same family as potatoes and tomatoes, so smoking should be avoided, although this did not apply to me, being a non-smoker.

Another appointment had been made for me in one month's time, in September.

By the time of the September appointment the symptoms of the candida had diminished somewhat, which was encouraging. The detoxifying tablets were helping to keep the arthritic pain and stiffness at bay to some extent; at night I could feel them working! They seemed to keep things moving inside, and I was feeling better in the morning than

Kathryn Lausevic

previously. But were they doing their job of cleansing the body of candida toxins?

Ralph began the testing, and yes...The greatest progress was the drop in the level of toxins – by two-thirds! This was good news and meant we could start hitting the candida in greater depth.

Another test showed that there was a considerable amount of protozoa, but this was not affecting me as much as the candida. Ralph affirmed that this could be eliminated within six months - more quickly if I adhered rigidly to the diet; and the less money I would need to spend!

Some foodstuffs were tested:- beetroot, soya milk and peppermint tea. All were found to be acceptable.

When we talked afterwards, Ralph stated that getting rid of the candida and protozoa were no problem. Then, when these were better, we could address the problems of the overpermeable mucosa - "leaky gut", the rheumatoid arthritis and the damage to the body.

He drew a graph to show how the toxin level goes up and down with the treatment. When you hit the candida the toxin level can rise dramatically so you have to treat it gently - not too much medication at first. Ideally the line on the graph should show a gentle downward slope.

With regard to joint deformities, for example the hands, he didn't see why these could not be improved, as the body completely renews all its cells in seven years. He remarked that if you care enough about improving these things, you can, even getting completely better!

I came out feeling very cheerful and decided to take a short walk in the woods. The sun was shining and the autumn colours of the trees looked beautiful.

At my next visit, on October 30th., the results of the tests bore out what Ralph had described on the graph. The candida level had dropped by half, but the toxin level had risen from two to five, on an arbitrary scale of 0-10.

Another factor which had contributed to the higher level of toxins was probably the fact that I had indulged in some foods which were not in my diet:- these included some delicious grapes, potatoes, red wine, coffee, (albeit "proper" coffee, which is supposed to be better than decaffeinated,) and some butter on a small piece of raisin bread. I had really been rather remiss, and had to remind myself that the only person who suffers from this sort of laxity is myself!

Could the results have been caused by a combination of these, or by preservatives/insecticides on vegetables and saladstuffs? Or maybe both....

At this visit the discovery was made that I was deficient in an enzyme which helps to digest food. This deficiency can cause undigested matter to leak through the intestinal wall into the bloodstream, causing joint pain and rheumatism symptoms. When the toxin and candida levels were *right* down we could address the problem of "leaky gut." I was looking forward to that!

As the candida leaves the body, it is advisable to attempt to replace the harmful bacteria with beneficial bacteria. This helps to balance the intestinal flora; one way to facilitate this is by taking "live" yoghourt.

Normal commercial yoghourt is made with non-human bacteria acidopholus. Ralph advised that human-based bacteria is obviously preferable as it is compatible with our existing bacteria and enzymes, so he suggested making my own yoghourt, with Bio-acidopholus, used in soya, sheep or goat's milk. The milks should be rotated. So I decided to "have a go" at that.

By November both the toxins and candida were further reduced and the protozoa had disappeared altogether. This was good news, and meant that I was practically ready to begin some new treatment to treat the remaining candida more effectively and to restore the acidopholus and bifidus. A human-based remedy would be preferable. Ralph had one in mind but when he tested me through Sandra, he found that I was intolerant to the herbs in it. Several others were tested but we could not find one I did not react to. He therefore decided to leave it for a fortnight, researching it in the meantime.

In December I was again tested for a suitable remedy to balance the intestinal flora and a suitable one was found, - Wild Pansy.

The morning previous to my appointment I had woken up with a great deal of pain, and experienced the worst day for several months. On deliberating about the possible cause of this I thought it might be *toothpaste*. A friend of mine, a dentist's receptionist, had obtained some new toothpaste for me and I wanted to try it, as it was recommended for keeping teeth white. (Mine were rather discoloured due to the daily vegetable juice.) I bought the small tube in the hope that it might achieve a minor miracle.

I had started using the toothpaste two days before my kinesiology appointment. The same day I started with a "flare-up" reaction, which gradually increased in severity during the next day. So the toothpaste was prime suspect and I took it to Ralph to be tested.

I sat with the toothpaste in my left hand, the other hand lightly placed on Sandra's right hand. Ralph pressed on Sandra's leg and nothing happened, -it resisted. Then he placed a magnet on the upper leg and pressed again. Nothing happened. He repeated the procedure, with the same result. Then he remarked, "It is a major allergy."

With some surprise, I remarked, "But the leg didn't move!"

He replied, "The muscles have become hypertonic (too strong). When I place the magnet on the leg it causes the muscles to weaken and therefore the leg goes down when I press. But the leg doesn't press down in spite of the magnet. It means that the muscles have become too strong - the opposite effect from the usual one, and this can indicate a major allergy."

Ralph also remarked that some kinesiologists do not always test in this way, and could regard the possibly allergenic substance as being "all right."

Before Christmas, I was dismayed to find that one of the remedies had ceased to be effective; this was the detoxifying one, which had made me feel more comfortable inside, and had a cleansing effect on the body.

For a while I seemed to have a regressive period, - a lot of pain and stiffness; this lasted about six weeks, right into February. This I connected with the lapse from the detoxifying remedy, as well as doing extra artwork at home; physical activity involving the arms usually had a detrimental effect on the body.

However, at the end of February it was found that the detoxifying remedy was now all right for me, as was also the one for the dysbiosis in the intestines. It was a relief to be able to take these again, and very soon I started to feel better.

Then, in March, the day I was hoping for arrived at last! The test for candida showed negative. So we could begin the treatment for overpermeable mucosa, commonly known as "leaky gut."

This condition is caused when the candida changes its fungal form, developing hyphae (sort of tendrils) which break through the intestinal wall, causing leakage of substances into the bloodstream. (See Appendix -"Candida.")

I had been looking forward to this treatment for a long time and felt very glad to be able to get to grips with it.

At the same session Ralph tested me for meridian imbalances and could find none. He remarked that he could not remember this ever happening previously, usually there is an imbalance of one sort or another, but I was perfectly balanced! I felt sure that my meditation practice had something to do with this.

The following tests in April showed that there was still no candida present nor were there any protozoa. However there was still a considerable amount of "leaky gut". As well as continuing the medication for this, I determined to fast for one day each week, to give the treatment a better chance to work, without any hindrance of food matter in the intestine or colon.

During the testing, an interesting incident occurred.

I was holding a phial bearing the words "rheumatoid arthritis", and because It affected me quite badly Sandra's arm muscles had become hypertonic (too strong), so that it was difficult for Ralph to test additional medications I might need. Ralph found a way round this problem and the muscles went weak. Suddenly the arm muscles went strong again! Ralph asked me, "What are you thinking?"

"I was thinking of eating a sandwich in Oxfam for lunch." I replied.

"What kind of sandwich?" he asked.

"A salad sandwich, but I was wondering if I could eat the bread."

"No, you can't!" he replied.

Bread contains gluten and previous tests had shown this substance to be unsuitable for me. Incredibly, even just my thinking of bread had affected Sandra's arm muscles!

Although this had been specifically checked by testing for a gluten allergy, it could have been that the stress of not eating bread for several months was enough to send the muscle hypertonic. This is an example of how Kinesiology sometimes can tell if there is a problem, but not necessarily what that problem is.

By July the leaky gut was considerably reduced, to my relief, and also the dysbiosis. But I had an excess of oestrogen. Why was this? Ralph then tested the liver - both parts, and found a problem in both areas of the liver; congestion, and poor liver function. It would be the liver congestion which was causing the excess of oestrogen, as the liver processes and recycles this hormone.

The congestion was probably due to improperly digested food, which would then create toxins which go into the bloodstream, causing "allergy" problems - joint and muscle pain and stiffness!

So I was prescribed a herbal remedy, and given a liver diet sheet to follow.

To be honest, I felt a little dubious about the findings concerning the liver. I had no reason to suspect that there was something wrong with the liver, except that I sometimes felt a pain in that area, which I put down to having undergone a gall bladder operation some years previously.

Then I remembered that eighteen months previous to the incident, an acquaintance, who does Shiatsu and Energy Balancing tested me and remarked that there was an "imbalance on the liver meridian." So this tied up!

At that time I seemed to be having a reaction after eating almost *anything*, except when I had detoxified myself. After detoxification my body was like a barometer for chemicals, pesticides and other unnatural foods such as refined sugar. I could tell in a very short time that *something* was affecting me, sometimes it was more difficult to find out what it was.

At the next Kinesiology session, in August, there was good news! Ralph could find no dysbiosis. So that meant that I was now clear of candida, leaky gut and dysbiosis, although the liver congestion was still present and I was to increase the remedy to six capsules per day. Also Ralph suggested now taking a medication which supports the adrenal glands; this would help to give me energy. At the same time he advised me that as the adrenal glands would be more active, if I felt any stress, anger or other strong emotion the best thing to do would be to express it, as suppressing feelings could cause the hormone to turn toxic in the body. This advice connected with what David Cousins had advised me to do several months earlier, - that I should laugh, shout, cry and scream if I felt like it! (See Chapter 9).

During our discussion Ralph gave me the following advice:- to follow a predominantly *alkaline* diet, at the same time keeping to the Liver Diet. I should also embrace Food Combining principles. (See chapter on Compatible Eating.)

At the next session everything went well. The liver was somewhat better, and Ralph now suggested a remedy which would help to rejuvenate it. This could be taken when the liver was sufficiently improved to allow it to work to optimum effect; there is no point in taking it before, as it would be like pouring water into a leaky pond. First you have to do the repair work!

I came out feeling "on top of the world."

Since my last visit, the pain in the liver area has almost disappeared; only occasionally does it make itself felt, and I can honestly say that most of the time I feel so *well*.

However, I have to be careful not to eat more sweet foodstuffs than is good for me. This causes a return of the candida to be dealt with once more. So my body is really saying that I should preferably avoid eating sugar or anything containing it, for the rest of my life, I suppose!

More recently, I have had Kinesiology sessions with my daughter, a well-qualified Kinesiologist who lives in Newcastle-upon-Tyne. She often tests me for imbalances such as mineral or vitamin deficiencies, or sensitivities to suspected foodstuffs. She also treats people with all kinds of disorders, such as problems from childhood; she also treats children with behaviour problems,etc. Her details are at the end of the book.

****

In June, 1997, I had a liver test, through a nutritionist, which still showed imbalances. The result showed a state which occurs as a result of exposure to endogenous or exogenous toxins, cigarette smoking (I don't smoke), certain medications or excess alcohol consumption. This we could not understand, as I hardly ever take any alcohol. So this remained a mystery, until I happened to see a recent programme on television, the subject of which was "Dysfunctional gut syndrome", the symptoms of which sounded very like candida.

A particular condition was described, which is called "Autobrewery Syndrome". In this condition sugar ferments in the body to alcohol. Immediately I thought of my liver test result (an excess of alcohol). Was the imbalance caused by still consuming sugar occasionally in the form of the odd cake or two, or a helping of jam, or even fructose in fruit and/or some vegetables? Sugar and/or yeast aggravates the condition so I would have to be more disciplined in my diet, in spite of having a sweet tooth. There is a book on the subject:-"The Autobrewery Syndrome", by J.Howard.

Both of these conditions, Dysfunctional gut and Autobrewery syndrome are caused by imbalances in the intestinal flora. There are no reliable clinical tests at the present time.

Foods recommended for these conditions were leeks, onions and garlic, which contain sulphur compounds, as well as probiotics, as found in "live" yoghourt.

After the liver test result I also had been advised to eat sulphurous foods including the onion family, cabbage and other cruciferous plants, eggs, meat and Epsom salts. However, as I had been advised to avoid onions and garlic, I eat them sparingly. A sulphur supplement is M.S.M., which I now take regularly.

CHAPTER 9.
ACCESSING ENERGY

In March,1995 I attended a workshop in London, run by David Cousins, the author of "A Handbook for Light Workers," which I had purchased about two years previously, as the title sounded relevant to the spiritual work I do each morning.

In fact it was no coincidence that I should be there; the previous year while on an artweek in Devon I met a lady who held David's day courses in her home in London. So I booked myself in. There is no such thing as "coincidence" anyway; all these synchronistic things that happen to us are just stepping-stones in our evolution towards discovering ourselves and our true purpose in life.

It was to be a momentous day. There were about fifteen people present, sitting in Ginnie's comfortable lounge on a cold March Sunday morning. David, who is an extremely psychic person, is a gifted clairvoyant. He told each of us many things about ourselves, which were also recorded on cassette for us to take home.

Some of the information channelled to me was "mind-boggling" - and gave me cause to take stock of my life.

Apart from certain personal disclosures David told me ways of helping my physical condition through meditation.

He gave me two specific meditations which I should practise several times each day.

The first one was to bring light into my body, by imagining a sun in each hand, a sun in each foot and one in my heart, then expanding this light with each breath to fill my whole being, until I was full of a wonderful bright, shining light.

The other meditation he gave me to do was to imagine the body as transparent. Starting with the skin, you have to look at any problems or blemishes, - any scar tissues, moles and so on. Then you breathe light into the skin until it becomes transparent, translucent...until you can see right through it to the flesh underneath.

Then you have to imagine going into the flesh - into the muscles, the veins, arteries and ligaments. You breathe in the light , concentrating on any painful areas such as painful muscles, until all the flesh becomes transparent and you can see right through it to the organs of your body.

Next you concentrate on the organs - first the eyes, ears, nose, then the organs of the main trunk of your body, the heart, liver, kidneys, etc. Then you breathe in the light as before, concentrating on any problem parts, until all the organs of your body become transparent, filled with beautiful light, and you can see right through them to the bones underneath, the skeleton of the body.

You then go into the bones of the body; first the joints, filling them with beautiful sunlight, breathing it in, once again concentrating on any problem areas.

Then you go into the bones themselves, actually into the bone marrow, filling with light, until all the bones become transparent. You do this until you feel that all the bones are completely translucent.

So then you are completely transparent, filled with beautiful, white, shining light.

After this you build yourself up again. First you see the bones return, but without any problems you had previously; then the organs appear....the flesh...and finally you replace the skin. See all your body return, but in a perfect state, without any problems at all.

I was advised to do these meditations five times a day! David also said that I would be completely well, and move into a "whole new space and a different tempo."

I was also told to express my feelings and emotions - shouting, singing, crying and laughing.

At first when I did the visualisations nothing much happened, except that I felt a beautiful sense of peace and calmness, which was my usual euphoric state during meditation.

However, after a week or two, some quite powerful things began to happen. When accessing the light my hands began to feel really heavy and numb. I visualised the light coming from my hands, up the arms to the painful places and spreading throughout my shoulders; it felt very good, relaxing and healing.

When I visualised the sun in my heart I saw it very bright and strong, and really felt that my heart centre was opening up, expanding... I was filled with love, total love and compassion for my friends, family,...for everyone. I felt I had unseen helpers; I seemed to be in a flow of Universal energy, which gave me an agreeable sense of balance and peace.

This feeling of harmony and connectedness also made itself evident in my everyday life. An example of this was if I was searching for something I would find it straight away. But there were obstacles too, - little pin-pricks and jolts to the ego and the patience, to see how I would react. I realised it was all part of a process.

And the healing began to work! I could do it anytime, - just had to "plug" into the Universal energy and let it flow through me, by visualising the sun...then bringing it into myself. So I gave thanks for this gift, this wonderful, free, accessible power which was helping me.

The revelations came almost daily. One day the realisation came that God is not "out there", He/She/It is in *me*. I had the power to make myself better. We pay thousands of pounds on medicines and help, and all the time the healing comes from WITHIN. Because God is in me, every action is sacred, every thought, every word, every deed SACRED. So we must do everything with great *care,* loving what we are doing. This means *flowing* with everything, not getting tensed up or stressed out, just taking everything as it comes, one thing at a time, gently and easily.

At the same time as I was doing the healing meditations I was releasing pent-up feelings. If I was angry about something I would go into the bathroom where no-one could hear and have a good shout and/or cry. This releasing always brought renewed energy and a release from physical pain.

Two months after the London visit another extraordinary thing happened.

This occurred at another workshop, this time a local one, "The Art of Living in Peace", run by David Keith, a wise, enlightened man who has done a lot of caring work on all sorts of levels in the Sheffield area.

A friend of mine, Carole, a Yoga teacher, happened to be there as well; she had heard about the workshop only the previous evening and spontaneously decided to attend.

At the workshop there were all sorts of interesting activities as well as information on the many aspects of peace, including some visualisations.

One of the visualisations was to imagine yourself small, then to "go into" a bone of your body. I went into the right knee, as it was the most painful place in my body. I just stayed inside, looking at the wall of bone.

Afterwards we went round the group, discussing the experience. Carole spoke before me and described how she had "gone" into her right knee. "But I don't know why!" She said she was "cleaning it."

I said,"I think you tuned in to me, because I went into my right knee; that is where I have the most pain." We just sat and looked at one another.

The next day I noticed that the knee felt better - the pain was hardly noticeable, and the knee was now better than the left one.

I phoned Carole and we decided to try the meditation on the left knee, the next morning at 8 a.m. We chose eight o'clock, as the number eight is the symbol for infinity, an extremely spiritual number and made up of two circles.

The next morning I awoke at two minutes to eight and jumped out of bed, giving myself palpitations in the process! I lit a candle and started the meditation, which lasted about ten to fifteen minutes. When I stood up at the end of the meditation, I realised, with wonder and joy, that the pain, which had been especially strong in the tendons behind the knee, had disappeared. In my diary that night I wrote, "I have *no* pain in the knee today - the first time for years! Yippee!"

Both Carole and I have read and been influenced by similar Spiritual teachings over the years, also we are both born under the sign of Pisces and it may be one of the reasons that we seem to resonate on the same wavelength. Out of the whole group at the Peace workshop, who else would be chosen but Carole, with whom I had so much in common, a compassionate person who would persevere and take the task of healing seriously. I cannot help but feel that the Universe had a hand in sending her to help, when my spirit was perhaps flagging a little and I needed some encouragement in the process of working with the healing energies.

After this Carole and I worked on different parts of my body in turn - the muscles of the arms, the elbows, shoulders, and other problem areas, with considerable success. One day I wrote in my diary:-

"Yesterday Carole and I concentrated on the shoulders, first the right and then the left. They were *both better* all day and right into the night, as was most of my body, except the right deltoid (always a problem), and the hips which were pretty 'bad' later on, and elbows."

In the evening of that day we had visited Alex's parents for a meal. Most of the food had been all right for me. I was very tired during the evening, so tired I could hardly keep my eyes open. We left and I had a shower then went to bed at about 10.15 p.m., after phoning Carole.

In the night the whole of my left shoulder started to ache -as bad as it ever had been, and there were other places in my body, which we had "healed", -left knee, arm muscles. I was so dismayed - was it failing? What had I done to cause this?... Then I remembered the RED WINE! I had drunk about one-and-a-quarter glasses full, mixed with spring water...but it hadn't been a very good quality. In my diary I wrote:-

"I realise how important and *sacred* is the work that we are doing. I must stay in a space of PURITY, of mind and body. It is a SACRED PRIVILEGE and I must not *abuse* it." So I asked my Guardian Angel for help, apologising for my carelessness.

The aches and pains disappeared and now I was determined to take more care.

One week later I wrote:-

"Have not had any severe pain all week, but the hips are a bit 'iffy', especially later in the day." But then I started doing a yoga exercise to help them, (lying on the back with the knees bent, lifting and lowering the pelvis), and since then they have been somewhat better; lying on the stomach is good, too, especially if you have had hip replacements.

Basically, though, I felt better generally. One day I worked on the computer for about three hours, with hardly any pain in the shoulders, arm muscles or hands.

The knees were incredibly pain-free, except a slight pain in the right one, on the inner side. It was wonderful after all the pain I had suffered with them, for many years...

The meditations had been done faithfully each morning, and at other times when I had a little space. It felt important, in fact as important as anything I had ever done in my life.

The wonderful thing about it is that the improvement is maintained, but only if I do the healing meditations regularly. If I miss doing the practice for a few days, my condition begins to deteriorate. So the Universe is intending me to keep my nose to the grindstone! But it is no hardship; I love doing it; it has become a necessary part of my life, especially more recently, as other developments started to happen...

At home I was experiencing some difficult personal problems. The only way I could cope with all this was to constantly put myself in the light. It was as though David Cousins had foreseen what was in store for me, and so had given me the Light meditations to practise. It never ceases to amaze me how the Universe provides for your needs.

Over the next few months I continued to bring the light into my body as often as was possible; even concentrating on it when I had a few spare moments in the day. It had become so important to me, manifesting a powerful effect on both mind and body. At the same time I was using affirmations to help me with the enormous personal challenges I was facing. For those people who are not familiar with affirmations, they are words or phrases of a positive nature, which, when regularly repeated, help to change one's thinking and attitudes.

As well as helping on a psychic level, affirmations played a large part in my physical progress, I believe. I spoke or wrote them almost every day. This practice, once again, owes its usefulness to the power of the mind. The repetition of words or phrases instils them into the subconscious and we can reprogramme ourselves to change our thinking and attitudes, accept new concepts and empower ourselves in any way we choose. If I had negative thoughts I would remind myself:-

THESE THOUGHTS ARE ALL IN MY MIND,
- AN ILLUSION. WHAT IS THE REALITY?
MY LIMITATIONS IN THE BODY
AND MIND ARE OF MY OWN MAKING.
THEREFORE I CHOOSE TO CHANGE,
LIVE IN THE MOMENT AND ENJOY EACH
MOMENT IN CENTREDNESS AND ATTENTION.
THIS SETS ME FREE.
EVERYTHING IS EASY BECAUSE I AM FREE.

Other examples of affirmations, which are written in my notebook, are as follows;-

I FORGIVE MYSELF,
THEREFORE I CAN FORGIVE OTHERS.
I LOVE AND ACCEPT MYSELF EXACTLY AS I
AM, THEREFORE I LOVE AND ACCEPT OTHERS
EXACTLY AS THEY ARE.

I AM A COMPLETE, WHOLE, INDEPENDENT
HUMAN BEING, WITH THE POWER TO
MANIFEST ALL MY DREAMS AND HOPES.
I FLOW WITH THE UNIVERSAL ENERGY.
I SURRENDER MYSELF TO THE UNIVERSE.
I SURRENDER EVERYTHING.
I AM A FREE SPIRIT; I AM FREE.

The word "surrender" implies *giving up* something or someone, - a detachment, a loss of dependance, of expectation even, as well as a detachment from negative feelings, such as resentment, fear, anger or anxiety. Sometimes I would release feelings by crying, when no-one was around.

I began to feel very free, empty even. It felt good.

****

Since this chapter was originally written, several years ago, it has become easier and easier for me to access the energy, causing a considerable healing effect on my body. Realising that if I can help myself in this way, in January, 1997, I joined the National Federation of Spiritual Healers as a probationary member, with the intention of helping others.

WHATEVER WE SEND OUT
COMES BACK TO US.

I would just like to add one thing. *Anyone* can access energy, with practice. Acquiring this ability brings responsibility, for it can be used for good or ill. The energy should always be used with LOVE and COMPASSION for all, unconditionally and without reservation.

As well as healing at close proximity, the energy can also be used for absent healing, that is, healing at a distance.

Even thinking about someone in a loving positive way is a prayer which helps their well being, for you are sending them energy. Even more powerful is to send a strong beam of light like a laser beam, from your solar plexus centre, and/or hands, to the person who needs healing.   Before you do this, however, you should always obtain the permission from the person who is to receive it. It is not necessary to obtain permission if you just "hold" a person in the light.

If you are interested in this work, some training at least in basics is advisable, and there are numerous books on the subject, such as Barbara Ann Brennan's excellent books, "Hands of Light" and "Light Emerging".

PART 2.
HOLISTIC SELF-HEALING –
BODY, MIND AND SPIRIT

CHAPTER 10.
COMPATIBLE EATING

Why was it, I asked myself, that sometimes I would eat a certain food, then afterwards suffer pain and discomfort, while at other times I could eat the same foodstuff with impunity? I was still asking myself this question in the summer of 1995.

A clue to solving this puzzle had arrived at Christmas, several years previously, in the shape of a little book entitled, "Food Combining for Health," by Doris Grant and Jean Joice. It was all about the Hay Diet, which I had heard of, but knew little about. At the time I received it the allergy testing was in full swing, so the book was shelved for the time being. Now, however, Ralph's remark about food combining had reminded me of it, so it seemed like a good time to see what it was all about and maybe put it to the test.

The principle of the diet, to put it very simply, is not to eat starch foods with protein or acid fruits, in the same meal. Foodstuffs fall into three categories:- "starch" foods, "protein" foods and "neutral" foods, the last of which may be combined with either starch or protein.

Of course there is a lot more to it than that, but that is the basic concept.

Many people had testified to the healing benefits of this way of eating, "not mixing foods that fight," and reports of the results include:- healed ulcers; digestion pain eliminated; improved arthritis and relief from rheumatism; freedom from constipation; relief from insomnia; depression changing to optimism, and freedom from colds. A woman of seventy had written, "I feel well for the first time in my life!" There were many more testimonies.

The diet was devised many years ago by an American doctor, Dr.William Howard Hay, who was born in Pennsylvania in 1866. A qualified doctor, he practised medicine for sixteen years, before becoming very ill with Bright's disease and high blood pressure which led to a dilated heart, whereupon he decided to change his eating patterns. He began to "eat fundamentally," - only natural foods, and in quantities suitable to his present need. Over the next three months his symptoms gradually disappeared and he felt fitter and stronger than he had for many years. He also lost about fifty pounds in weight, and as he had been considerably overweight this was a great bonus.

Dr. Hay's experiences with this method convinced him that medicine was on the wrong track, attempting to remove the symptoms rather than the cause of illness. He made no claims to "cure" a disease, emphasising that his system "merely removes obstacles in the way of nature's marvellous healing powers."

His ideas were met by disbelief and scepticism by the medical profession in general, who were not ready for these untraditional concepts, especially as the new "wonder drug" era had begun. Dr.Hay died in 1940, a year after a serious accident.

Since then there has been a change in attitude to nutritional value in disease, and it is now a priority in preventive medicine.

Dr. Hay claimed that the causes of most degenerative diseases are connected with food, the culprits being over-consumption of refined carbohydrate, and incompatible combinations. It is now agreed by many doctors that the over-consumption of refined carbohydrate is responsible for the degenerative diseases, which are different manifestations of this one cause. This concept is known as "The Saccharine Disease".

Most allergies, too, are caused by a deranged body chemistry connected with the food we eat and how we eat it. A secondary cause is from irritants to the system such as pollen, smoke, certain substances in food or foreign proteins (natural irritants).

The authors of the book maintain that arthritis is a purely nutritional state, therefore the logical treatment is a nutritional one. This exciting and thought-provoking concept signifies hope for the alleviation of symptoms for the arthritis patient, bringing relief from pain, possibly after many years of suffering.

When the body is relieved of excess debris, and the diet is corrected, Dr.Hay claimed that even severe cases of arthritis can recover, even when there is immobility, with pain in every joint, although deposits in the tissues round the joints may take years to be reabsorbed into the body.

The factors listed in the book which contribute to arthritis include:- injuries to the body, e.g. overuse of joints or muscles (especially in osteoarthritis); allergic reactions; infections; stress.

The main common denominator of these factors is that the chemistry of the body is incorrectly balanced; there is an excess of acid and a lowered reserve of alkali. Research has shown that our body chemicals are naturally in the balance of 80% alkaline and 20% acid; therefore ideally this is what we should take into ourselves. This means that our alkaline intake of food should be four times greater than our acid intake, for optimum health. In his book, "Foods for Health and Healing," Dr.Dudley d'Auvergne Wright observes that the normal alkaline state of the body fluids is the most favorable one for the action of vitamins.

Indigestion is common in arthritis, as there is often difficulty in assimilating carbohydrates. If this is the case, it is helpful to eliminate starch and sugar. If the separation of different types of food is strictly observed, it is claimed, no other treatment is necessary in many cases, especially if a mainly alkaline diet is followed. A high intake of acid fruits is recommended to help the body's alkaline reserve. Of course all diets are subjective and as I have already emphasised, you may find that you are affected by certain foodstuffs and these are obviously best avoided.

The reason why starches and sugars should not be eaten with proteins in the same meal is that alkaline-forming foods and acid-forming foods require different conditions in the stomach for their proper digestion. Proteins require an acid medium for digestion; if the meal is a mixed one of proteins and starch and/or sugar, the protein is incompletely digested. Furthermore, the starch content of the meal, which needs a positive alkaline medium for the digestive process, will not be properly broken down and digested, therefore causing fermentation and indigestion. This also happens when starch is eaten with sulphurus foods such as peas, beans, cabbage, cauliflower, Brussels sprouts or eggs, or with foods containing acid, such as citrus fruits, vinegar and tomatoes.

When proteins are not properly digested, instead of splitting up into amino acids, they form large protein molecules which are actually toxic. Some of these molecules make up the substance known as histamine, a well-known toxic protein which is potentially the cause of hay-fever, asthma and other symptoms.

What is histamine? In my dictionary it is defined as follows:- Histamine is a white crystalline compound, the action of putrefying bacteria. It stimulates *gastric secretion,* contracts smooth muscle, and is released during allergic reactions.

So histamine is connected with acid build-up. And acid build-up causes stiffness and pain!

Histamine is normally destroyed by a healthy liver, but a damaged one, as I have, has difficulty in dealing with it. The plot thickens! (More about histamine in Chapter 17.)

Like Dr.Hay, Arnold Ehret, in his book,"The Mucousless Diet Healing System", stipulated that a mixed meal is acid-forming, and acidity is a sign of disease. High protein foods decompose very quickly when mixed with body gases and cause acids and toxins. We need only a small amount of protein. Ehret declared that fruit, the food which is poorest in protein, provides the body with the greatest energy and stamina. And acid, of course, causes internal discomfort.

This information was of particular interest to me personally, as many years ago, when in my thirties, I had continual discomfort in the stomach and bowel area, which the doctor called "gastritis", prescribing tablets which I took for many years. I was thinking about this recently, then I remembered Auntie Connie.

"Auntie Connie", my father's sister, who died about thirty years ago, had a great many stomach problems when she was young. This, I think, was the main reason why she became vegetarian, even actually opening a vegetarian guest house in a suburb of Bournemouth. A vegetarian guest house was quite an innovation in those days, the 1940's.

Of course, being a vegetarian would cut out a lot of potential problems connected with acid-causing protein such as meat, thus enabling Auntie Connie to live a full, comfortable life which she subsequently did for many years.

Ehret, then, maintained that diseases are connected with mucus and toxins in the stomach, intestines and mostly the colon. He claimed that rheumatism and gout are caused by mucus, and by uric acid accumulated in the joints. He declared that physical treatments, including massage, exercise, breathing exercises and osteopathy can never heal properly without proper attention to diet.

Even the wrong sort of cooking can be acid-forming, as well as destroying healing nutrients. "Wrong" cooking includes boiling in too much water, and also frying. (See Chapter 11 -Diet and Vitamins.)

A food researcher in Germany, Ragnar Berg, proved scientifically that every food which contains mucus after decaying produces acid at the same time. So if you eat acid producing, mucus-forming foods such as meat, dairy produce, nuts, eggs and starchy foods, you should compensate by eating a large number of fruits, vegetables and starchless green vegetables (alkaline foods) in order to be healthy.

Both Arnold Ehret and Dr. Hay advised eating as much fresh, raw, whole food as possible. Raw foods, being high in fibre, relieve constipation and cleanse the intestines. These foods are rich in potassium, which is a powerful alkaline substance. Both Arnold Ehret and Dr. Max Gerson believed that disease begins with an imbalance of sodium and potassium in the body. Usually there is too much sodium and too little potassium, especially in the western diet. If the balance is corrected by eating potassium-rich foods such as fruits, salads and raw vegetables, the cells of the body are re-vitalised and made more efficient in fighting disease; this applies even to cancer. Fatigue can be caused by a deficiency of potassium as also can high blood-pressure.

In arthritis, the action of potassium dissolves and disintegrates deposits of minerals such as lime and chalk, which cause stiffness and pain. Potassium also helps to keep the heart, arteries and bloodstream free from clots and calcification, which causes increasing disability. Salt (sodium) has the opposite effect from potassium and therefore should be reduced to a minimum. In cooking, the use of herbs will help to flavour the food.

Fruits with the greatest amount of potassium include bananas, avocados, blackcurrants, melons, kiwi fruit, pomegranates and rose hips.

Vegetables high in potassium include the green-leafed ones, especially broccoli, spinach, water cress, parsley, cabbage, kale and fennel.

Recommended Foods - Alkali-Forming.

Salads, all vegetables, including jacket potatoes if the skins are eaten, (but please see Chapter 11 for ones not recommended for arthritis); all fresh fruits except plums and cranberries, almonds, seeds, such as sunflower seeds, sprouted seeds, soya products.

Acid-Forming Foods - Not Recommended!

All animal proteins, fish, shell-fish, eggs, cheese, butter, margarine, lard, poultry, nuts (except almonds), peas, beans, lentils, all starch foods such as cereals, grains, bread and flour and other foods made of cereal starches, sugars.

"Acid-forming" refers to the end product in the body, not to the medium necessary for their digestion, which is acid for animal protein and alkali for starches.

Many people have a gluten problem, and some of their symptoms can be associated with sensitivity to wheat. Nowadays wheat is sprayed with pesticides and herbicides; this could be the cause of the intolerance, which may not apply to other grains, even though these contain gluten. Symptoms of wheat toxicity include heart problems, high blood pressure, anxiety, migraine and many gastro-intestinal problems.

To sum up compatible eating, then, according to the Hay System, there are five important rules:-

1) Starches and sugars should not be eaten with proteins and acid fruits in the same meal.

2) Vegetables, salads and fruit should form the major part of the diet.

3) Proteins, starches and fats should be eaten only in small quantities.

4) Only whole grain and unprocessed starches should be used. All refined, processed foods should be avoided, in particular, white flour and sugar, and all foods made with them, also highly processed fats such as margarine.

5) An interval of at least four to four-and-a-half hours should elapse between meals of different character.

This way of eating, that is, separating the different types of food actually dates back to ancient times, back to our roots! When we look back into ancient history, we see that primitive man did not sit down to a meal of meat and two or even three veg. First of all he would eat only when he was hungry. He would find a patch of something, maybe greenstuff, fruit, roots or berries, and eat only what his body required. Then when his stomach would tell him it was time for the next meal he would move on to something else. If an animal was killed for food this would constitute a meal on its own. So he did not mix his food.

Some other recommendations, especially for arthritis, by Dr. Hay include:-

1) Taking celery juice. (See Juice Therapy chapter.)

2) Taking wheatgerm, bran, kelp (sea-weed) and cod-liver oil.

3) The elimination from the diet of vinegar (I have always found this "lethal", and anything containing it, such as mayonnaise), spices, tea, coffee and alcohol, especially sweet wines and liqueurs.

4) Gentle exercise and natural sunlight.

5) Calmness and emotional control. Negative emotions such as fear, tension, anger or hate tend to exacerbate the symptoms and increase suffering.

When I started to put the principles of this diet into practice it wasn't long before I began to notice an increased feeling of internal comfort. The difference was more no-ticeable after meals, as foods which were compatible with one another were digested more easily. This in turn caused an improvement in general well-being, with less pain and stiffness.

To be frank, however, I have to say that I find it very difficult to eat like this all the time, especially when eating out at friends' houses, or in restaurants. So I do not rigidly follow the diet. But then, from time to time, I have come across several different preparations which have helped with this dilemma. One of these was perhaps one of the most important revelations in my marathon search for physical "healing." I discovered....Aloe Vera.

This product is described in the course of the next chapter....

CHAPTER 11.
DIET, SUPPLEMENTS
AND VARIOUS
NATURAL REMEDIES.

There is a definite link between rheumatoid arthritis and what one consumes. When an arthritic person changes their diet to one which is suitable for their condition, the difference to the amount of pain suffered can be quite dramatic. This is good news, for it means that the patient can help himself to a great extent, by modifying his diet and even by eliminating certain foodstuffs which aggravate the problem. If you are aware of the connection between the pain you suffer and what you eat, you have the opportunity to help yourself, if you so wish!

Inflammation is accelerated by certain substances which are contained in animal fats, i.e. red meat and dairy produce. Some other fats, which contain substances known as free radicals, lead to destruction of the joints. These fats include heated polyunsaturated oils. Reheated oils are particularly "lethal", so chips are not recommended, or indeed anything fried! Also bad for arthritis are hydrogenated fats, such as those found in margarine or packaged foods, so always check when purchasing.

You may be wondering what free radicals are. Free radicals are unstable oxygen molecules. Actually they play an important part in the body by destroying disease-causing bacteria. Usually they are kept in check by natural substances in the body called antioxidants, but if they get out of hand and proliferate they have a harmful effect on the immune system, and are thought to be the most common cause of cancer, auto-immune diseases, senility, memory loss, ageing and wrinkles.

How does this happen?

The cell walls of the body are made up of polyunsaturated fats, and when these are attacked by free radicals they turn rancid, (just as butter does when exposed to oxygen,) causing damage to the surrounding body tissue. In rheumatoid arthritis the damage causes excess fluids, swelling and pain.

So what causes the free radicals to get "out-of-hand?" The following external factors have been found to increase the amount of free radicals in the body:-

1. Excessive exposure to X-rays.

2. Radioactive contamination; this includes low grade radiation from mobile phones,microwave ovens, even computers.

3. Pesticides, colourings and other chemicals, industrial solvents and CFC's.

4. Pollution. This includes pollutants in food, water, cosmetics and drugs.

5. Smoking -passive and active.

How can we protect ourselves from an excess of free radicals?

Antioxidants are our best protection. They neutralize the potentially damaging effects and arrest the spread of free radicals, therefore preventing foods, especially fats and oils, from oxidation.

The most commonly recognised antioxidants are Vitamins A, B6, C and E, and beta carotene, plus the minerals selenium and zinc.

Vitamin A is found in dark green vegetables and fruits, also in eggs, milk, lamb's liver, halibut liver oil, cod liver oil, dairy products, pig's kidney, carrots, beef, mackerel and canned sardines. However, if too great an amount is taken Vitamin A can be toxic, as it is stored in the liver, so care must be exercised not to eat these foodstuffs in excessive amounts. The body's store of Vitamin A is protected and increased by Vitamin E so it is vital to have both in the diet.

Vitamin B6 (Pyridoxine) is beneficial for the synovial membrane, so important in rheumatoid arthritis, and helps to control pain and restore joint mobility. It also helps to metabolise proteins and fats. The main sources are potatoes and other vegetables, bananas, poultry and white fish.

Vitamin C (Ascorbic acid) cannot be manufactured by the body, so we have to depend on sufficient intake in the diet. Unlike other vitamins, it is required in large amounts which could only be supplied by an enormous amount of fruit and vegetables such as those found in tropical regions. Scientists think that at some point in history we lost the ability to manufacture Vitamin C in the body.

Many diseases could be connected with this fact as almost everyone is deficient in this vitamin. A high level of Vitamin C indicates a low risk of heart disease and certain types of cancer. According to Patrick Holford, author of "Say No to Arthritis", the optimal amount to reduce these risks may be at least 500mg. a day. But for arthritis patients 3 to 5 grams a day is recommended.

Not only does Vitamin C help to synthesise collagen, the intercellular "glue" which keeps all our organs, muscles, skin, tissues and the digestive system intact, but it protects against pollution of the body by toxins, carcinogens, free radicals and heavy metals. Energy cannot be made in any cell without adequate Vitamin C. For people suffering with arthritis, it is essential in assisting the formation of healthy collagen for bone and cartilage, and for the body's formation of natural cortisone.

Vitamin C plays a large part in boosting the immune system. Being anti-viral and anti-inflammatory it is powerful in fighting infection. A recent test has shown, in the test tube, that it can even inactivate the HIV virus.

Foods containing Vitamin C include citrus fruits, green vegetables and potatoes. In fruit it dissipates quickly when exposed to the air. Even the action of squeezing the fruit destroys the vitamin. Ascorbic acid can be added to foods but it can cause some discomfort. Probably the best way to take Vitamin C is by taking buffered supplements, with at least 4% bioflavonoids (beneficial nutrients).

Vitamin D helps to control the calcium balance in the body. Together with magnesium and calcium it strengthens bones and joints.

Sunlight is a good source of this vitamin as the light converts certain chemicals found in the skin, into Vitamin D. This may be one reason why people with arthritis feel better in the summer. People who are not exposed to enough light are usually deficient in this vitamin.

Foods rich in Vitamin D are meat, fish, eggs and milk. People who do not eat these foods may need a supplement.

Vitamin E has many important functions, some of which are as follows:- it protects lipids (fats) in the cell walls; increases exercise capacity; stabilises membranes; protects muscle tissue and prevents tumour growth. It is enhanced by other antioxidants including Vitamin C and the mineral selenium. In fact the combination of Vitamin E and Vitamin C is thought to reduce inflammation and speed up the healing of joints, as together they help to synthesise mucopolysaccharides, a natural lubricant for joints and component of cartilage. Vitamin E is found in oils, e.g. wheatgerm, safflower, sunflower, soya bean; nuts and seeds, spinach, asparagus, broccoli, butter, bananas and strawberries.

Beta Carotene has a powerful effect in destroying free radicals, therefore it is important to have an adequate amount in the diet. Foods containing beta carotene include spinach, carrots, broccoli, kale, peaches and apricots. It is extremely safe to take. The only possible side effect occurs when taking high levels. This is a yellowing of the skin and will pass when the high dosage is discontinued.

Supplementing the diet with zinc can be very beneficial for rheumatoid arthritis patients, as it helps to reduce the pain and swelling. It also helps to facilitate the proper digestion of proteins, which, if not properly digested, can cause allergies which lead to joint inflammation. Together with Vitamins A and C, zinc is needed to keep the wall of the intestinal tract strong and healthy, as a common problem with rheumatoid arthritis is an overpermeable intestinal wall, which allows unwanted substances to leak through into the bloodstream. (See Chapter 17.)

Zinc is found mainly in cheddar cheese, beef and stewing steak, bread, eggs and chicken. In vegetarian diets, seeds such as pumpkin, sesame and sunflower contain zinc, but in grains and legumes there is a substance called phytate which binds up the zinc so it is not so accessible to the body. For vegetarians then, zinc supplementation in the form of capsules may be needed.

Calcium is the most abundant mineral in the body, 99% of it being found in bones and teeth. People with arthritis need a good supply of calcium, especially post-menopausal women who are more prone to osteoporosis. However, it cannot be used properly by the body without magnesium. Low magnesium levels are associated with osteoporosis. An adequate intake of calcium, Vitamin D and magnesium, among other nutrients, increases bone density.

Another thing which increases bone density is regular exercise on the weight-bearing joints, such as walking. This can increase calcium levels by 2%.

A high calcium intake will not be beneficial if you are taking too much protein, as protein foods are acid forming, and a high protein diet leads to calcium deficiency. No amount of calcium will counteract it. Some medical scientists now believe that a high protein diet is a primary factor in osteoporosis.

In his book, "Say No to Arthritis," Patrick Holford writes that dietary calcium intake is only one of the factors which influence the proper use of calcium in the body. There is a whole list of factors which negatively affect this delicate balance, most of them connected with diet and lifestyle.

Sources of calcium include milk, cheese, natural yoghourt, sardines, tofu, watercress and dried figs.

A trace element, boron, found in soil, food and humans is also required to prevent calcium loss. Tests have shown that supplementing with boron improves symptoms in a few weeks, in 80-90% of cases. A supplement can be obtained which combines calcium, magnesium and boron.

Selenium is a mineral which has several vital functions in the body; it prevents degeneration of liver tissue, protects against cancer, maintains a healthy heart, and inhibits the harmful effects of heavy metals such as mercury, cadmium, arsenic and lead. A deficiency of selenium is often found in areas where the soil is poor in this mineral. The main sources of selenium are meat, particularly organ meats, fish and shellfish, plus wholegrains and cereals. Sesame seeds and sunflower seeds are high in selenium, Vitamin E and calcium, as well as zinc.

Before taking large amounts of these nutrients, it is necessary to be aware of the following facts.

I quote from "Vitamin Guide", P.22:-

"The immune system can be both strengthened and weakened by dietary intake of nutrients. Optimal intake of vitamins A, C, and E and the mineral zinc will strengthen the immune system, increasing resistance to colds and more serious infections, but larger daily doses actually suppress the immune system. This is because the immune system includes several feedback mechanisms which recognise higher than required intakes. Consequently the system 'slows down', to cope with the increased intake."

There are so many minerals, vitamins and trace elements which are vital to a healthy body that perhaps vitamin and multi-mineral food supplements may be the best form in which to take these. But extra Vitamin C is usually needed, and other supplements may be required. For pregnant or lactating women it is not advisable to take supplements without medical supervision.

In order to take the right supplements, with the correct dosage for your particular case, the best thing to do would be to consult a qualified nutrition consultant, who will advise you and give you a comprehensive programme to follow.

If you experience any adverse reactions when taking supplements, it is best to stop taking whatever you suspect of causing the reaction, and consult a qualified nutritionist or doctor.

Fish oil

The essential fatty acids found in fish oil are anti-inflammatory, helping to reduce the symptoms of arthritis. These fatty acids, commonly called EPA and DHA cannot be manufactured by the body, so are a desirable part of the diet of an arthritic person. Fish rich in these oils include mackerel, herrings, sardines, fresh tuna, trout and salmon. Many people take the oil in the form of capsules; however some of the capsules are very small so it may be preferable to take the bottled variety, (Cod liver oil or Halibut liver oil,) as it takes several capsules to make up the optimum requirement.

"Vitamin Guide" states:-

"The use of fish oil concentrates on sufferers of rheumatoid arthritis has been shown to reduce the symptoms of swollen and tender joints, morning stiffness and pain."

There is a word of caution about fish oils. Patrick Holford states that both fish oil and aspirin thin the blood, so it is not advisable to combine both of these on a regular basis.

Some Natural Remedies

Rheumatoid arthritis is an immune-related disease, so anything which strengthens the immune system is all to the good.

Two herbal remedies which help the immune system are *echinacea* and *quercetin.*

Echinacea, derived from a plant, is excellent for stimulating immune activity, and is used by American Indians as a snake-bite antidote! These are its properties as a remedy:- It is anti-viral, stimulates immune activity, enhances white blood cells very quickly and increases interferon - a protective protein.

Quercetin is also anti-viral and is a natural pain-killer cum anti-inflammatory agent, so is especially useful for rheumatoid arthritis. It also speeds up the production of collagen which is a primary component of cartilage. Quercetin should preferably be taken between meals, as it works better on an empty stomach. It is found naturally in onions, broccoli, squash and red grapes.

DLPA

This has proved to have a most dramatic effect on the amount of pain I have had, in spite of discovering it only recently.

DLPA was described in two separate sources which came my way, as a substance used for pain control; it is also used for depression. When I mentioned it to a friend with arthritis she lent me a book on it!

DLPA stands for DL-phenylalanine and is a nutritional amino acid (not a drug). It works by protecting the endorphins, the body's natural painkillers, which also influence our moods. One of the "side effects" is that it increases your energy level! I have found, since I started to take it that I need less rest and have increased enthusiasm and energy.

The amount of endorphins the body produces is affected by *stress*, e.g. continual physical pain and emotional upset . With fewer endorphins available the amount of pain increases, so it is a vicious circle. Many people suffer from a stress-induced lack of endorphins . Moreover the body also makes certain enzymes which "chew up" the endorphins! This depletes the supply even further. What DLPA does is to slow down the activity of these attacking enzymes, thus allowing the endorphins to do their pain-blocking work and increasing their lifespan.

Another effect of DLPA is as a powerful, safe antidepressant. It has been proved in clinnical studies to be as effective as antidepressant drugs.

DLPA is non-addictive, has no side effects and is non-toxic to humans.

When you begin taking it you may not see any effects for a few days, even for several weeks. But my experience showed a marked improvement in a very short time. When you have a whole pain-free week you can stop taking it until the symptoms reoccur - this may be as long as two to three weeks.

Evening Primrose Oil.

This natural oil is known to have remarkable health giving properties, due to the fact that it contains an unusually high content of gamma linolenic acid (GLA), which is a dietary necessity for a healthy body.

Another substance which has remarkable healing properties is Aloe Vera.

Aloe Vera

I came across Aloe Vera through one of those inexplicable "coincidences" which have dogged me for the last ten years. At Unstone Grange, a lovely Victorian mansion in Derbyshire, which is used as a centre for all kinds of events, courses and workshops, and where I sometimes help in a voluntary capacity, we held a Women's Nurturing Day. The treatments on this day included Massage, Reiki and Reflexology among others; I decided to have a Reflexology treatment. The practitioner was a knowledgeable and perceptive man called John, (not his real name,) who told me something about Aloe Vera and actually sold it for a well-known national company. From his recommendation I decided to try it.

John described the wonderful healing powers of the juice which is obtained from the Aloe plant; this juice is used to help relieve all sorts of conditions from A to Z, including asthma, bronchitis, irritable bowel syndrome, digestive problems, haemorrhoids, infections, insomnia, liver and kidney ailments, M.E., rheumatism and arthritis, sore throats, thrush, ulcers, and varicose veins; these are only some of the whole list compiled by Paul Hornsey-Pennell in his book, "Aloe Vera, the Natural Healer". (See Bibliog.)

The Aloe Vera ("true" aloe) plant looks like a cactus, with long, fleshy leaves ending in a point. Inside the leaves is the jelly, which contains the healing properties. These properties include antibiotic, growth stimulating, pain-killing and coagulating potencies.

The use of Aloe Vera in medical practice dates back 4,000 thousand years to the ancient Egyptians and it was also used by the Greeks and Romans, as well as in China, India and Persia. Down the centuries it has spread throughout the world.

In modern times Aloe Vera has been used in the treatment of radiation burns after early use of X-rays, and also for survivors from nuclear explosions in the 1940's. Examination of people treated with Aloe Vera revealed inexplicable healing, tissue growth and reduced pain and scarring.

The resulting interest in this plant inspired research to be carried out in the U.S.A. and Russia, but however much it was studied, although its main constituents were discovered, no-one could ascertain the secret of its healing powers.

I do not propose to go into too much detail about Aloe Vera as you can read about it in a specialist book, such as the one I have mentioned. But here is a list of some of its impressive properties:-

Aloe Vera contains Vitamins A, B1, B2, B6, B12, C & E. There is not space here to say what the function of all these vitamins are, but you can find out what their properties are in a good vitamin book, such as "Vitamin Guide". (See Bibliog.)

The minerals which Aloe Vera contains include calcium, chromium, copper, magnesium, zinc, sodium chloride and potassium.

The healing properties of Aloe Vera include the following:-

Antibiotic, anti-inflammatory, virucidal, and bactericidal, antipuritic (relieves itching), and antipyritic (relieves heat associated with burns and inflammation). It is also excellent for the skin, softening and moisturising.

Aloe Vera used for Detoxification

Aloe Vera causes increased absorption of nutrients into the system, as it softens waste matter such as caked-on mucus, so that it is more easily eliminated, therefore cleansing the intestinal tract. This enables food to be better assimilated and processed, which in turn causes better functioning on all levels.

The potassium contained in Aloe Vera stimulates the kidneys also in ridding the body of waste matter.

In testing Aloe Vera on patients with a variety of conditions, the vast majority reported that they felt an increased feeling of well-being, felt happier, with more energy, and were sleeping better. Their symptoms had improved from "slightly" to "dramatically", with the time taken for the effects to manifest varying between an instant response, to several months, depending on the individual and the nature of the problem. As for myself, I began to notice certain improvements after taking the juice for two or three weeks. I realised with delight that I could eat some foodstuffs which had previously affected me badly, without any serious repercussions. The feeling of tiredness during the daytime became less, and I suddenly realised one day that the fatigue which had been a constant companion for many years seemed to have faded away - I had more energy and stamina, even being able to do activities like gardening, standing and bending, without any after-effects. I even felt able to plan whole days out, as previously there had been some anxiety that I might be too tired "on the day".

As Aloe Vera is not a drug, you have the choice of how much to take. Up to four tablespoonfuls a day is the recommended dose for arthritis. It is usual to take two in the morning, and sometimes two in the evening, depending on one's condition.

Sometimes you may feel worse before feeling better; this is because the juice is flushing through the system, exposing any problems and disposing of toxins. After a few days this should settle down.

When buying Aloe Vera it is always best to check the ingredients. Some time ago I purchased a bottle by mail order and after taking one dose there was a reaction of increased pain. On reading the small print on the side of the bottle I saw that it contained preservative. Needless to say *that* company lost a customer!

Another helpful product, which contains Aloe is Swedish Bitters. This preparation performs a similar function to Aloe Vera in maintaining a comfortable and regular digestive system. As well as Aloe, it contains mainly extracts from herbs and roots, and like Aloe Vera it provides the missing bitter element in our diet, balancing the sweet, salty and sour food which constitute the bulk of a normal diet of a western person.

Swedish Bitters is quite expensive, but you only need a small amount - one teaspoonful at a time, after a main meal. It is really useful if you have eaten something which "disagrees" with you, or would cause indigestion or other problems. For me, it has the same effect on arthritic pain reactions as Aloe Vera does. During the Christmas period I found it absolutely wonderful in regulating the digestive system, thereby preventing reactions to food from which I would otherwise have suffered.

Glucosamine Sulphate

This preparation was recommended to me some years ago by a nutritionist, a well-known practitioner in Sheffield.

Glucosamine sulphate protects against joint destruction. It also provides relief from arthritic pain and inflammation, thus enabling the patient to avoid taking aspirin or other NSAIDs (Non-steroidal Anti-Inflammatory Drugs), which although they suppress the symptoms, have been linked with increased joint destruction.

Glucosamine, which is found naturally in cartilage, stimulates the production of substances needed for joint repair, so as well as protecting the body against damaged joints it helps the body to repair joints which have already been damaged by arthritis.

Glucosamine sulphate is an amino acid attached to a sugar molecule which is in turn attached to a sulphur molecule. This breaks down quickly in the body, as the molecule structure is relatively small. Glucosamine sulphate has proved to be very safe, with no attributable risks or side-effects.

Tests have shown that the longer it is taken the greater the benefits; one study, which compared glucosamine sulphate with Ibuprofen, showed that although it takes longer to produce results, after four weeks the group receiving glucosamine sulphate were significantly better than the group taking the drug.

Glucosamine is one of the substances which has allowed me to eat a greater number of foodstuffs, some of which affected me previously.

Vegetarian Glucosamine is also available.

There is another source of help which I must mention.

One of the possible causes of arthritis is thought to be connected with infections. Sometimes viruses and/or bacteria lodge in the joints, recurring when the natural immunity is below par. (See Chapter 17 - The Causes of Rheumatoid Arthritis.) Instead of taking prescribed antibiotics, which can exacerbate or even eventually cause thrush and candidiasis, there is a product which has been discovered only relatively recently, which, like Aloe Vera, is a natural antibiotic.

(For further information on treating parasitical infections please see Appendix 3.)

Grapefruit Seed Extract. (Citricidal)

This was discovered fourteen years ago by a gardener who was also a doctor and a physicist. He noticed that when he threw grapefruit seed onto his compost it did not rot down. Upon investigation he discovered that the extract made from the seeds was an effective anti-microbe with remarkable properties. Since then it has proved successful in the treatment of many disorders and conditions.

As well as being able to inactivate viruses, yeasts, fungi, parasites and worms it is also efficient in the treatment of sore throats, flu, gingivitis, diarrhoea and food poisoning. It is highly effective for treating skin conditions such as athletes foot, warts and acne.

The advantages of grapefruit seed extract are that it is natural, inexpensive and non-toxic; above all, while being lethal to the harmful bacteria, it does not seem to disturb the beneficial microbes.

Grapefruit seed extract can be successfully used to treat chronic candidiasis; this condition is often linked with rheumatoid arthritis as it can cause gut permeability.

Many medical practitioners are now prescribing grapefruit seed extract for candida.

It has also been successful in the treatment of secondary infections in AIDS patients.

As grapefruit seed extract is extremely strong it should always be diluted in water or juice. It should not be used in the eyes, although it may be used externally on the skin, as a mouthwash or nasal rinse, or mixed with glycerine for ear infections. Maybe we should all have some in the first-aid box.

Other supplements which have been useful are Slippery Elm and Psyllium Husks. Both of these are excellent for the digestion. Slippery Elm facilitates the process of the food in the gut and makes you feel really comfortable inside, and Psyllium Husks prevents constipation by providing bulk to your diet.

RECENT DISCOVERIES

Since this book was first published, in fact very recently, I have discovered two supplements which have proved to be remarkably successful for arthritic pain.

The first is called **Samento.** Another name for it is Cat's Claw (Uncaria Tomentosa). It has been used by the indigenous people of Peru for centuries. This natural remedy is now being used in more than forty countries worldwide.

Samento's natural properties act on the cellular immune system. Most species of this plant, Uncaria Tomentosa, contain another group of actives which inhibit the beneficial action. These alkaloids are called TOA's . Samento, however, is certified to be 100% TOA free.

Researchers in Austria have carried out tests on people with rheumatoid arthritis, and found it to bring significant relief from painful and swollen joints, and to reduce morning stiffness.

Samento can also be used for Chronic Fatigue Syndrome, MS, Parkinson's disease and Lyme disease. It can be safely combined with most medication, but is not recommended for those with an allergy to Quinilone based antibiotics. It is also not recommended prior to transplant surgery or for those who have undergone transplant surgery, because of its immune boosting properties.

Another supplement I have recently found helpful is **Serrapeptase.** This is a proteolytic enzyme known as the second gift from silkworms. It offers powerful support for healthy joints, lungs, inflammation, arteries, veins and colon. I quote from the Naturally Health brochure. "Wonderful results with a variety of conditions have been reported in various studies and also by practitioners observation of patients." Serrapeptase is said to reduce cysts (such as cysts on the ovaries) and scars. It is suitable for vegans as it does not contain any animal products. It is safe for everyone and there are no known side effects. It is suitable for any inflammatory condition. You can also use it for animals.

Both of these supplements have helped me enormously in the last year or so, since I started using them.Then about two months ago a friend told me of an interesting machine used by a local practitioner, at a clinic in Sheffield. She was looking for someone with rheumatoid arthritis to see if it would help the condition. I volunteered to be a "guinea pig!"

InterX 5000 Therapy

When Russian scientists were asked to develop a method of treating astronauts in space without using drugs, they invented SCENAR technology.

All water gets recycled during space emissions, even that which leaves your body, so it was important not to use antibiotics and other drugs, which would contaminate the water. SCENAR(self-controlled energo neuro adaptive regulator) devices took a different approach to the problem. The cells in your body communicate with electric signals and the new technology imitated these signals to allow a "conversation" with the body at cellular level. The body is then stimulated to release the neuropeptides needed to repair a problem and carry on releasing them even after a treatment session is finished.

After trials it was licensed to use in Russian hospitals in 1985 and today ambulances in Russia carry Scenar devices to treat casualties on the way to hospital.

This technology has now come to the West, where we benefit from the knowledge of the Russians' 20+ years of experience and trials. The latest devices are known as InterX 5000 and InterX is now a recognised therapy in the UK where it is licensed for pain relief.

Unlike TENS, InterX can stimulate your body to go beyond just blocking pain to addressing the causes of it and many acute injuries (including sports injuries) typically heal in a third to a half the time taken with other therapies. Biofeedback is given during treatment to elicit optimum points of treatment.

It is a pleasant therapy to experience as the device is small and treats by movement over the skin, both on problem areas and whole body treatment (especially on the spine, from which the nerves radiate to the rest of the body.) Where a site is too painful for treatment, treating the opposite side of the body can still produce the healing required.

When people who have tried other therapies for a problem (especially long-standing ones) come across InterX and remark they wish they had encountered it sooner.

Some of the conditions which have shown improvement with the use of InterX include sports injuries, recent or long term pain, muscle spasm, arthritis, whiplash, post-operative discomfort, back problems, digestive disorders, urological problems and phantom limb pain. It is also useful for stress relief and cosmetic applications which can be an aid to health in toning musles, promoting weight loss and improving one's sense of well-being with tonong of stomach muscles, thigh, buttock or arm firming and facial toning.

I have now had eight treatments and have a space of four weeks before any further treatment. This allows the body to absorb the effects, as the healing process continues during this time. However, I have been immensely impressed by the effects which I noticed, even after the first treatment. I have attended the clinic with a variety of symptoms over the last two months, including pain in shoulders, elbows, hands, wrists, arm muscles, in fact, typical rheumatoid arthritis symptoms. All these have shown improvement, in fact have mostly disappeared! It is quite incredible. Whether these wonderful results will last or not, it is too early to say. But I am cautiously optimistic.

THE DIET

For a person suffering from rheumatoid arthritis the diet, to a great extent, is subjective. It is a matter of trial and error - foods which suit one person may give problems to another. Generally speaking, however, the guidelines to diet given by the Arthritic Association are excellent ones to follow, and it is probably correct to state that certain foods, for example dairy products, affect most arthritic people.

All dietary advice should be treated with a little caution, until you have tested it personally. For example I am very fond of fruit. Now, on the list given out by the Arthritic Association in which points are ascribed for each foodstuff, apples, grapefruit, oranges and lemons are given low points which means that in theory they should be all right to eat, but I discovered many years ago that all of these fruits, especially citrus fruits, are pretty toxic to me, causing a lot of pain. At one time I was eating stewed apples and suffering some considerable pain. Suddenly I realised the implications; when I stopped eating the apples the beneficial effect was quite noticeable. Pineapples too have the same reaction. So it is always best to proceed warily.

Fruit, especially unpeeled, is also not recommended if you have a yeast problem, or a "dysfunctional gut" (See Chapter 17), because of the fungus (yeast) found on the surface of the fruit, as well as the fruit sugar. This applies also to vinegar, which is fermented, commercial juices, left-over food, and bread, which of course usually contains yeast, although you can now buy certain yeast-free types of bread.

The most common offenders in the diet are dairy produce and grains. Milk intolerance is very common in people with rheumatoid arthritis. Many reports have been published showing allergies to dairy products, in arthritis. Of course there are alternatives. Soya milk, natural yoghourt and rice milk are available, or goat's milk may be tolerated. There is also soya cheese or non-dairy cheese such as rice cheese.

Grains are extremely subjective; some people cannot tolerate oats or wheat. Wheat, in fact, is our number one allergen. It contains gluten, a gastrointestinal irritant, which is also found in barley, rye and oats. Some people also have a reaction to corn (maize). Grains which are usually tolerated are rice, millet, buckwheat and quinoa, a staple food from South America.

With regard to flour, there are number of additives used in the processing of it. Patrick Holford observes that not even a weevil can live on white flour!

Although most vegetables are tolerated by arthritics, there is some evidence to suggest that certain ones are not good for arthritis; these are the deadly nightshade family of plants, and include potatoes, peppers, aubergines and tomatoes. The tobacco plant also belongs to this family, so smoking has a detrimental effect on rheumatoid arthritis. Smoking also causes damage from free radicals. (It is said that one puff of cigarette smoke can contain up to 100 trillion free radicals!)

Caffeine in tea, coffee and chocolate causes certain protective fluids to be eliminated more quickly from the body, and alcohol, too, aggravates arthritis. It destroys the protective nutrients and disturbs beneficial fatty acids. It is high in calories and suppresses the appetite. In "Say No to Arthritis" there is a lot more information about the harmful effects of coffee, tea, sugar, chocolate, cola and alcohol.

In red wine and chocolate there is a natural substance called tyramine which some people are sensitive to; this is also found in various cheeses.

Many people find they cannot tolerate animal fats. These contain saturated fats which block the conversion of essential fatty acids into anti-inflammatory substances called prostoglandins. So it is preferable to avoid them.

I must say a word about meat here. It is a fact that the higher up the food chain one goes, the greater number of toxins are accumulated, as each "link" in the chain is absorbed into the living organism. So plant foods are safer to eat than animal products. Although this also applies to fish, from my experience I have found that the advantages of eating fish outweigh the disadvantages; it is an excellent source of protein as well as providing essential fatty acids.

Anything containing chemicals, colorings or preservatives should be avoided if possible. For myself I have found that they are one of the biggest factors in causing pain and stiffness. Patrick Holford declares that there are vested interests in keeping the general public ignorant about the nutritional deficiencies in most foodstuffs. Even the British Nutritional Foundation, which advises the government on nutritional policy, is funded by major companies producing confectionery, high fat foods, processed meats, food chemicals and alcohols.

So what can one eat and drink?

In describing my own diet, I have to say that it is fairly restricted as so many foodstuffs affect me. You will have to find out for yourself what you are able to eat. The proof of the pudding, as they say, is in the eating!

Apart from eating fish and occasional free-range chicken, I have found that a basically vegan diet works the best, with lots of alkaline foods, such as salads and vegetables.

My diet, therefore, consists of a myriad of vegetables of all kinds, preferably raw - fresh green leaf ones for the mineral content are especially useful; rice, both white and brown; avocados; oils - olive oil, safflower, sunflower and rapeseed oil; salads of all kinds except tomatoes and peppers; cereals including sugar-free rice cereal, oatbran and organic cornflakes, rice cakes, pumpernickl, sunflower seed bread and sprouted wheat bread (there are various ones on the market, one with ginger is especially good), multigrain gluten-free bread; many sorts of seeds including sunflower, linseed, millet, pumpkin seeds and sesame; quinoa; some nuts, especially almonds; fish of all kinds including tinned fish; beans of all kinds; soya milk and rice milk; occasional free-range poultry, and organic free range eggs. With regard to protein, surprisingly many "vegetarian" foods contain a higher quality of protein than that found in meat. These foods include quinoa, soya, peas, beans, lentils, nuts, seeds, grains and even some vegetables such as spinach and broccoli. The only fruit I eat is an occasional apple, which I often put in the juice.

As already mentioned, oily fish is excellent. These fish include mackerel, herring, salmon and cod. The fish should not be fried, as heated fat contains free radicals, which contribute to joint destruction. Baked or poached fish is delicious.

Oils should preferably be raw - cold pressed virgin olive oil is the best; it contains oleic acid which is especially useful if you have candidiasis. Other beneficial oils are safflower and sunflower. The fish and raw oils provide the body with certain anti-inflammatory fatty acids. Linoleic acid found in vegetables has the same effect.

Onions and garlic are beneficial in that they contain amino acids which are essential constituents of cartilage. Onions also contain natural quercetin which is anti-inflammatory.

If you do eat fruit, it should be eaten between meals, or perhaps half-an-hour before the main meal. This is because of the processes used in its digestion. Many people finish a meal with fruit but this is not as good for the system.

As detailed in Chapter 10, the best way to eat vegetables is in their raw state, and as fresh as possible. All food should be as natural and unadulterated as it is possible to be. I quote from Leslie and Susannah Kenton's book, "Raw Energy,"

"...remember that the further a food gets from its natural state the worse it is for you. Anything artificial or chemically processed is automatically suspect.... Here are some of the main offenders:- most convenience foods; frozen prepared foods; white flour and white bread, even packaged 'brown bread', white and brown sugars (not dark brown molasses sugar); coffee and tea; anything containing sugar (saccharin, glucose syrup, corn syrup, dextrose, etc.), preservatives, flavourings, permitted colour, emulsifiers, edible starch, stabilisers..."

In planning meals I try to maintain the principles of Food-combining as far as possible.

I usually start the day with some juice, made on the machine. This is excellent for giving you energy and provides you with some of your daily vegetables. (See Juice chapter).

For breakfast I either have an egg, usually boiled, with ricecakes or corncakes, or I eat some ricecakes with rice slices, which taste like cheese. Sometimes I have cereal, but instead of milk I have it with hot water or rice milk, which is delicious. With the cereal there are seeds such as sunflower, millet and linseed, ground up in a coffee grinder. These are excellent energy boosters. I also eat gluten free brown bread with hot water (pobs), to which I add almonds and soya yoghourt.

If I am at home lunch is usually taken at about 1.00 p.m. or later. In fact it is not a good idea to eat until you are really hungry! Only when you feel really ready for a meal can it do you the optimum amount of good, otherwise you may be overloading your system.

For lunch then I usually have a salad, made with as many raw ingredients as are available, maybe lettuce and/or rocket straight from the garden, cabbage finely chopped, watercress or land cress, grated carrot and/or celery, cucumber, beetroot and anything else available - perhaps some left-over cooked rice. With this I sometimes have some tinned fish - tuna, sardines or salmon, or perhaps an avocado. Lunch, however, is usually an "alkali" meal, especially if I have had protein for breakfast. Instead of bread there are rice cakes, sunflower seed bread or pumpernickl, which is made from rye, or I may have a jacket potato. For dressing I just use olive oil, sunflower or rapeseed oil. Afterwards I usually have some live soya yoghourt. Sometimes as a treat I have a little non-dairy or soya ice-cream.

I usually have my main meal at 6.30 p.m. or thereabouts. Sometimes I have a home-made vegetable soup, made with whatever vegetables I have in the house, usually bought fresh that day. If there is some cooked chicken that goes in as well. (Free-range of course.)

I usually prepare at least three different kinds of vegetables; there are many to choose from so I vary it considerably. I often have rice, or jacket potatoes or boiled new potatoes, or occasionally quinoa, a staple food from South America. When cooking rice I usually add seeds such as pumpkin, sunflower and/or sesame seeds. Roast potatoes for me are "out". The reason I don't eat pasta is that it is made with wheat flour, and I have a gluten problem. Chips, too, are "killers" because of the heated oil.

Occasionally I prepare beans, perhaps butter beans, haricot beans or a mixture of different kinds, which I cook with vegetables such as leeks, celery and carrots, adding a few herbs like sage or thyme. Sometimes I have an avocado with the meal; they are extremely nutritious.

A delicious way to cook "hard" vegetables is to steam them for ten minutes and then bake them in the oven in a dish smeared with a little cold pressed oil, for half an hour or more. This method converts the starch into fruit sugar and is very good for the blood. Vegetables which can be cooked in this way include celery, cauliflower, carrots, potatoes, leeks and parsnips, among others. Normally, however, if you *have* to cook vegetables the best and most simple way is just to steam them, for as short a time as possible. This retains more goodness than boiling them.

Salt should be used only sparingly, if at all, as it upsets the delicate sodium/potassium balance in the body. To drink, I usually have boiled filter water, as the chemicals in tap water affect me. Spring water is fine, but it should not be heavily mineralised; Malvern or Highland Spring are the best. Rice milk makes a refreshing drink; it can be purchased at health shops. With dinner I occasionally have a glass of red wine, which suits me better than white wine. It has been discovered recently that red wine contains quercetin, which has powerful anti-inflammatory properties, as already stated.

For myself, in spite of some limitations in what I eat, I enjoy my food enormously. This, I feel certain, is due in part to the nature and taste of pure, fresh and unadulterated food (as far as it is possible to know). When you have eaten in this way over a period of time, you become very discriminating about what you put into your body. You begin to look at every food for its value in energy, for instance, and for its purity; therefore most edible products you see in supermarkets are not even entertained as suitable foodstuffs for your body, which is, after all, the temple of the soul.

CHAPTER 12.
THE JUICES

"...a healthy body can only be built out of high-quality nutrition and pollution-free foodstuffs ".

- John Davidson,
"A Harmony of Science and Nature."

Fruit and vegetables contain all the essential nutrients we need, provided they are uncooked. They contain concentrated vitamins, minerals, trace elements, enzymes, sugars and proteins.

In disease we need to consume as much fresh, raw fruit and vegetables as possible. This provides our bodies with the high mineral and nutrient content we need for energy, the energy which helps to fight illness and enables us to cope with our lives more effectively. The best way to access large amounts is by making juice, on a purpose-built juice machine.

Taking juice rather than solid raw food places less strain on the digestive system, which is often an important factor for people who are perhaps not well anyway, or elderly. By making juice, which is easily assimilated, the nutrients are absorbed into the bloodstream almost as soon as they reach the stomach and small intestine.

By taking juice you can consume perhaps a half a head of celery, half a cucumber, two or three organic carrots, a beetroot or two and a mass of green leaves, all in about one pint of fresh, delicious-tasting juice.

Because of all the nourishment contained in them, the juices are excellent, not only for arthritis, but for other diseases and disorders. Some examples include:- cabbage juice for stomach ulcers; spinach, cabbage and nettle juice for anaemia; carrot and beetroot for allergies.

The green-leafed vegetables are full of chlorophyl, which is also beneficial for heart disease, sinusitis, pyorrhea and depression, among other conditions. Carrot juice aids the elimination of toxins, as well as increasing muscle tone and improving vitality, due to its high mineral and vitamin content.

Other diseases which can benefit from juice therapy include colitis, diabetes, multiple sclerosis and toxaemia. It is also excellent for people who have a weight problem, as it helps to control the appetite. A regular user will find it easier to maintain a healthy weight.

There are two vitamins which are toxic if taken to excess; these are vitamins A and D. Vitamin A is produced from carrot juice, but the amounts recommended in the books fall within safe limits. Vitamin D is found in cod liver oil, which, when taken to excess can cause toxicity.

Juices for Arthritis

One of the most important vegetables for arthritis is celery. It works as a cleansing agent, clearing away waste material. It also helps to maintain the correct consistency of fluids in the body, as it is high in organic sodium and organic potassium, which balance one another. It combines well with carrot juice.

The following suggestions are merely a guide to give you some idea of what
to put in the juice for arthritis; they may of course be varied according to what is available.

To celery juice you may add:-

Cucumber – 10 fluid oz; nettles 6 fluid oz.

Nettles – 13 fluid oz.; parsley – 3 fluid oz.

Spinach – 8 fluid oz.; parsley – 3 fluid oz.

Cucumber – 6 fluid oz.; beetroot – 7 fluid oz.; water-cress – 3 fluid oz.

Carrot – 10 fluid oz.; beetroot – 7 fluid oz.; cucumber – 3 fluid oz.

I am not suggesting that you weigh everything! This is just a rough guide.

These recommendations are based on the findings and experience of many natural healers and other therapists over many years. However these suggestions are for guidance only; you can be quite creative in your juice-producing efforts.

The amount of juice you take should ideally be at least one pint every day, although less than that will also have a beneficial effect. Obviously the greater the amount you take, the greater the benefits you will feel.

The juices play an important part when fasting, as they supply vital nutrition to keep the body energy high, without the encumbrance of solid food matter.

Preparation of Vegetables

The fruit and vegetables should be raw, of course, and organic if possible, especially carrots which more easily absorb pesticides and pollutants from the soil. If you can grow your own produce so much the better, but if this is not possible, the best available foodstuffs should be used. As soon as a plant is picked the nutritive value begins to decrease, so freshness is an absolute priority. With regard to the green leaves, almost any edible green leaves are suitable. I sometimes come in from the garden bearing dandelion leaves and nettles, as well as broccoli leaves, radiccio, spinach or lettuce.

When preparing the vegetables and fruit, they should be washed well, before cutting into pieces which will fit the hopper of the juice machine. It is best to use filter water to wash them, as the chemicals in the tap water may affect the arthritis.

The juice should be drunk as soon as possible after preparing as the precious energy-giving enzymes decrease fairly rapidly. Enzymes are produced by living cells and help to accelerate the numerous reactions which take place in the digestive system, so that cells can function properly. They are protein and are destroyed by heat (over 54 C).

Juice Machines

There are many different kinds of juice machine on the market, which vary in price as well as in efficiency. Once I had a very expensive American one, which was extremely efficient, but you needed considerable force to push the vegetables into the hopper; so it actually aggravated the pain in my arms and shoulders! Needless to say, I didn't persevere with it for very long, as it was so counter-productive.

The one I use now, although it may not be the best on the market, is a centrifugal type juicer, which is easy for me to use. However, the drawback to this type of juicer is that it does not extract the maximum amount of juice, leaving the pulp moist rather than dry. In order to obtain the maximum amount of juice, I remove the pulp after juicing, then put it through the machine again. This breaks up the fibres and extracts additional juice.

If you intend to make juice it is advisable to purchase a book on the subject. There are many different ones, which can be obtained at healthshops or bookshops. A good book will give you instructions for making the juice in addition to information on the various fruits and vegetables recommended for different medical conditions. Even if you have no specific health problem, the juice gives you wonderful vitality, keeping you in peak condition!

CHAPTER 13.
VARIOUS HELPFUL THERAPIES

"The cure of the part should not be attempted without treatment of the whole. No attempt should be made to cure the body without the soul and if the head and the body are to be healthy, you must begin by curing the mind. For this is the great error of our day in the treatment of the human body, that physicians first separate the soul from the body."

- Plato.

Holistic therapies are now widely used and accepted almost everywhere. These are ones which treat the whole person. They are increasingly popular, as more and more people are now realising that we are a whole entity with mind, body, emotions and soul. If one or another of these parts is impaired in any way, then treating another part in isolation is virtually useless; there may seem to be a temporary improvement but long-term problems will still remain, and even the patient may not understand the reason.

Many practitioners combine different treatments according to the needs of the patient. Some therapists use herbalism, dietary advice and/or counselling, among other therapies. Some people have emotional problems which inhibit their progress, perhaps causing them to retain negative feelings such as resentment or fear due to past circumstances. They may benefit from counselling, psychotherapy or hypnotherapy sessions. The mind is extremely powerful in contributing to the causes of disease, and it is well-known that even events which happened during childhood can have long-term effects and prevent us from being in the right harmonic frame of mind for any sort of healing to take place, whether it is physical, emotional, mental or spiritual. It is therefore imperative to sort this out before anything else, in order for other therapies to have any effect in the long term. There are many books written about the power of the mind in healing; without a doubt it is an immensely important factor, if not THE most important.

When healing takes place in the mind, the whole body comes into harmony, which then allows natural healing processes to manifest. However, other therapies are often needed and there are many helpful ways to combat pain and discomfort.

A common problem in rheumatoid arthritis is the presence of localised painful areas, places in the body where there is tenderness and soreness. There are a number of things you can do to help ease this pain, to bring relief.

One very simple way is the application of hot or cold compresses; most people prefer one to the other. A hot water bottle or heated pad may be placed on the affected part for those who prefer heat; others may find a cold application more effective. Bags of frozen peas can be used, as already mentioned. The advantages of this is that they are accessible to everyone, and the peas move about and settle satisfactorily onto the area. If the peas feel too cold, the packet may be placed inside another bag, or be wrapped in a tea-towel, then applied to the sore place for about twenty minutes or so. Simple, but effective! After use it can be returned to the freezer for further use, in fact the same bag can be used many times.

Another way to help ease the painful spots is by massage or aromatherapy, which usually provides considerable relief. A visit to a trained practitioner is wonderful of course, but if you are having a distressful spell, with discomfort every day, frequent visits would be inconvenient as well as formidably expensive, so a little massage at home may be possible, as well as extremely beneficial. The help of a husband/wife/partner might be co-opted, or someone else may be prepared to give up ten or fifteen minutes in the day to help you.

Preparation for Massage

The room should be quiet, private and warm, with no interruptions such as the telephone. If using the floor, a sleeping-bag or futon will be needed for lying on; pillows for supporting areas of the body, some towels, and some massage oil if required. There should be enough space round the person being massaged for ease of working.

The towels will be needed for covering parts of the body, and also for the "patient" to lie on, especially if using oil. They may previously be placed on a radiator in readiness. It is extremely comforting to be covered by soft, clean, warm, fluffy towels. A bath sheet is good.

If you are having the shoulders or back massaged, you should prepare to lie on the floor or on a couch, in a prone position (face down). This is preferable to sitting on a chair as the weight is taken off the limbs and is supported by the floor or the couch.

First of all, take off any thick clothing such as sweaters. Ideally all clothing which covers the area to be massaged should be removed, in order for the treatment to be most effective. The person being massaged might prefer to undress in private, in which case a large towel is useful to wrap around the body; the natural modesty of the patient should be respected.

When the person is lying down, pillows may be used to support different parts of the body for comfort; it is obviously supremely important that the person should be as comfortable as possible. As well as a pillow for the head you might like to place one under the lower legs for support. Then the towels are used to cover the "patient"; the area to be massaged should be the only one to be exposed; towels may be placed over other parts of the body.

All that your partner needs to do is to kneel down beside you and find the affected places, the most painful spots, with your guidance, pressing the fingers or thumbs into these tender areas, holding and releasing. This usually brings much relief. Often your partner will discover the places to massage, as "knots" can be felt, small lumps which move under the fingers. Your massage partner will soon come to learn where the tender spots are.

If he/she is using oil, the oil bottle should be within easy reach as it is distracting for the "patient" if the "masseur" keeps moving away to pour out some more oil! Ideally the person doing the massage should keep in continuous contact with the person being massaged; even when moving round the body it is pleasant to keep one hand on the person's body as reassurance.

The amount of pressure involved is entirely subjective. Sometimes you may prefer a greater pressure so do not be afraid to communicate this to your partner.

Other massage techniques which may be tried include:-

(1) Stroking ("effleurage"); this has many uses including locating tenderness, tightness and spasm; deep pressure of upward strokes provides a passive stretch to the muscles.

(2) "Kneading," as though you are making bread; this, among other things, helps to disperse toxins from the muscles and oxygenates the tissues. It also helps the flow of blood back to the heart.

(3) Friction: small, penetrating circular movements; this is useful for massaging deeply into joint spaces and breaking down hard muscle knotting, nodules and so on.

Holding is very effective as it is calming and nurturing to the receiver. At the beginning and end of the "session" it is a useful and therapeutic exercise just to place one's hands gently on the patient's body; on the shoulders or head maybe. In fact as well as being soothing to the receiver it gives the "practitioner" the opportunity to "tune in" to how the patient is feeling and make reassuring contact with them.

If the person being massaged has a heart condition, it is stressed that great care should be exercised. Only gentle massage is advisable in this case.

There are other massage techniques and a good book on the subject will describe them. All the techniques can be combined as desired. There are some important factors to remember, however:-

(1) Always massage towards the heart.
(2) Never massage an inflamed joint.
(3) Do not massage the spine, which is extremely vulnerable and may be damaged.
(4) Take care in massaging painful areas and be prepared to stop if there is too much discomfort for the patient.

You may like to give yourself a massage, as long as you can reach the painful parts! This can be effective, even without removing any clothing. It may be tried on the shoulders, neck, arms, hands and fingers, legs and feet. You could massage your hands while watching television, or even sitting with family or friends. If you are not confident about self-massage a qualified massage practitioner will give advice, and show you simple techniques and exercises to do at home. Practitioners are generally very helpful and pleased to pass on information.

The use of massage oils is both pleasant and beneficial, as the oils are absorbed through the skin and into the bloodstream, therefore going straight to certain organs of the body. There are two types of oil which may be used:-

1) A base or carrier oil. There is a whole range of these, including sunflower oil, grapeseed, sweet almond, soya oil or plain vegetable oil. Some of these can be purchased in the supermarket.

2) Essential oils. These can be added to the base oil, and as well as being attractive by virtue of their scent they are used for different purposes, according to what is needed.

For example, some may have a relaxing effect, while others are stimulating.

A word of caution is needed here. The essential oils contained in massage oil should be used with care, as each of them has specific properties. Some can even be harmful to certain conditions. There is a whole list of hazardous oils, and another list of ones which should be used only with caution. An example is that Rosemary is not recommended for people with high blood pressure or epilepsy. Certain oils should be avoided during pregnancy, and care should be exercised with the elderly and also with young children. If unsure, check with a qualified aromatherapist.

An increasingly popular form of massage is Shiatsu. This is an oriental art form of therapy, as is the more commonly known acupuncture. Both of these ancient systems of healing work on the energy channels of the body to restore harmony and balance, which has a profound healing effect on the whole body. The energy channels, called meridians, nourish the vital organs and the practitioner works on points on these channels, the energy centres. In acupuncture the needles are placed at these points to correct imbalances, or remove energy "blocks", thereby restoring the balance of the "chi," the life energy, to create a sense of harmony and well-being. Pain is usually relieved in varying degrees, sometimes temporarily but quite often permanently, or at least for some considerable time.   Acupuncture is effective for a wide variety of conditions, through its power to stimulate our own healing responses. In addition to arthritic and rheumatic aches and pains, other disorders which can be helped by acupuncture include anxiety states, asthma, depression, back pain, skin conditions and many others.

Shiatsu works on the same principle, that "chi," or energy is transmitted via the meridians to all the organs of the body. Through the skill of a practitioner the whole body is nourished and revitalised, leaving a wonderful sense of peace and well-being. Elaine Liechti, in her book "Shiatsu," suggests that choosing between Shiatsu and acupuncture treatment is a matter of individual preference and upon health condition. Some people like the nurturing feeling and closeness of Shiatsu, while others prefer the less intimate approach and distance of the acupuncture needles. Some practitioners who use both give acupuncture for acute, painful conditions such as arthritis, frozen shoulder or any kind of blockage or severe pain, while Shiatsu is administered for chronic persistent conditions which need long-term rebalancing, maybe at a deeper level. Indeed, both of these therapies are recommended to bring relief. Acupuncture is an exacting and beautiful art, very successful in the hands of a skilled practitioner, while Shiatsu is extremely relaxing and psychologically beneficial as it gives you a delightful "pampered" feeling!

"The power of compassionate touch is immense. The power of healing touch, used with a knowledge of energy in a system such as Shiatsu, has the ability to enhance people's lives in a tremendously positive way. By reaching out through Shiatsu and improving the quality of individuals' lives we can perhaps improve the quality of Life for everyone upon our Earth."

- Elaine Liechti,
"Shiatsu - Japanese Massage for fitness and health."

Other complementary therapies include Homoeopathy Chiropractic, Reflexology, Kinesiology (see separate chapter), Biofeedback, Alexander Technique, Feldenkrais Method,

Polarity Therapy, Gestalt Therapy, Flower Remedies and many more. It is not within the scope of this book to describe them all, but I must mention one or two that I have found to be particularly helpful.

Chiropractic impressed itself on me when I had a knee problem, as already described in another chapter. The right knee was "locked" for five days and I was unable to walk or even put my foot to the ground. On friends' recommendation I went to a Chiropractic Clinic for treatment, during which the chiropractor managed to straighten the offending knee. So I walked out of the clinic pushing the wheelchair in which I had arrived!

In "Alternative Medicine, a Guide to Natural Therapies", Dr. Andrew Stanway gives the definition of chiropractic as, "An entirely manipulative therapy designed to maintain the spinal column and nervous system in good health without the use of surgery or drugs."

The use of chiropractic dates from ancient times. There are descriptions of chiropractic techniques in ancient Egyptian manuscripts. Manipulative treatment was also used by the ancient Hindus, Chinese, Babylonians and Assyrians. Somehow it fell into disuse, only being "resurrected" in 1895.

Its modern use and understanding is based on the work of Dr. Daniel David Palmer, a Canadian, who cured his janitor of deafness by manipulating his neck. Being encouraged by this he undertook further study of anatomy and physiology, eventually evolving the philosophy and treatment known as chiropractic.

In the past, chiropractic was not well-regarded by the medical profession in general, as many doctors did not accept or recognise that some health problems can be caused by slight deviations of bony parts, especially in the spinal column, which cause interference in nerve transmissions.

Now, however, the reputation of chiropractic has grown, and it is the most widely recognised worldwide complementary medicine. Chiropractic students train full-time for four years, studying many subjects which doctors do, but with a special emphasis on the spine.

How does it work?

First the chiropractor takes a short history of the patient's health condition and problems.

Often X-rays are taken from which the chiropractor can work, ascertaining the state of the spine and other joints, and where the problems are.

Joints are manipulated by hand in order to restore the function of the body. Usually the spine is treated, but the treatment may be given to any areas of the body. The aim of the treatment is to correct postural distortions, restore reasonable function to spinal and pelvic joints and to remove any nerve irritation which is causing pain or disturbed function.

As well as manipulating the joints, the chiropractor may give advice on diet, exercise and rest, and sometimes advise other treatments, such as massage, heat treatment or yoga.

In arthritis, many cases can be helped if they are not too severe. If there is joint destruction, however, the response may be small, but some relief may be obtained if the dysfunction of the joints is able to be improved.

Other conditions which respond well to chiropractic include low back pain, slipped discs, neck, shoulder and arm pain, and some surprising conditions such as asthma, migraine and even indigestion!

It is important to make sure that the chiropractor is properly qualified, as there are some dangers, but in skilled hands the treatment is very safe; in America the insurance premiums of chiropractors are lower than those of physicians or surgeons!

Reflexology is an extremely useful therapy for arthritis. Areas of the body which are too painful to be massaged can be reached by massaging the appropriate places on the feet. The definition of reflexology given in "Alternative Medicine, a Guide to Natural Therapies," by Dr. Andrew Stanway is:- "An ancient Chinese and Indian diagnostic and therapeutic system in which the soles of the feet and less commonly the palms of the hands are massaged deeply."

The reflexologist presses the feet to locate sites of crystal-line deposits which tell him where the problem areas are in the body. He can diagnose which organs are affected by disease or other problems. The patient feels pain in the area pressed on the foot and also in the associated part of the body.

The treatment consists of pressure applied with the edge of the thumb or finger, rotating clockwise. It need not be painful, as a good reflexologist would rather give several short pain-free treatments than one in-depth painful one.

As well as being therapeutic for arthritic pain, I have personally found that reflexology helps in releasing toxins from the body. It is also extremely relaxing and nurturing.

The Alexander Technique is concerned with the use of the body, using it in the right way, changing bad habits of posture and thinking into ones which promote well-being throughout the whole self. It was devised by an Australian, Frederick Matthias Alexander, (1869-1955). Because he had problems with his voice (he was an actor), he started to observe himself. Through this self-observation he developed a system, which was to re-educate the body to be used in the correct way. The system includes exercises and breathing techniques. Now you may not think that this is crucial to your everyday living, but *how* we sit, stand and move are extremely important, not only for the body but indeed for the mind as well, which sometimes needs to change old habits and thought patterns.

Once the technique is learned it becomes an integral part of yourself, and has a transformative effect on your whole being. You become very *aware* of how you do everything, and seem to acquire a grace which will not permit you to adopt poor attitudes, both of posture, perhaps "slouching," or equally important, of the mind, (which perhaps has been "slouching" as well!) because when we are standing, sitting and moving correctly it gives us a wonderful sense of harmony, balance, order and freedom. Actors, singers and musicians are all well-aware of this and it is a joy to see a pianist such as Alfred Brendel play the piano sitting so beautifully on the stool, with such grace.

Glen Park's book on the Alexander Technique, "The Art of Changing," is extremely comprehensive, with helpful drawings and diagrams. In the words of the author,

"Whatever you do the technique can help the quality of your life to improve. It can help you to learn how to sit, stand, move, write, drive, think and feel in richer and freer ways. The technique is a foundation for living, and it comes to life by being applied to the daily activities of life. It offers both a mental and physical approach to all activity, and a method of bringing about changes which can be applied to all aspects of life."

Nowadays there are numerous therapies available and often different ones are used for different purposes according to a person's needs at a particular time. He or she may sometimes require one sort of treatment and sometimes another, depending on the problem. However, it is now generally accepted that negative states of mind can prevent the natural healing processes of the body to do their work, as already mentioned. One of the ways these problems can be addressed is with the use of Flower Remedies. The best known of these are the Bach remedies, but there are others. The flower remedies all work to correct imbalances on subtle levels, on the principle that states of mind such as fear, worry or resentment inhibit the vital flow of healing energy throughout the body, which eventually can even produce disastrous effects which cause disease.

The story of how Dr. Edward Bach evolved the flower remedies is a fascinating one. It is described in "The Medical Discoveries of Edward Bach, Physician." (See Bibliography). The healing properties of flowers have long been recognised. The remedies incorporate the elements of earth, air, fire and water. When being prepared they are placed in a glass bowl filled with water, then placed in the open air on a sunny day. It is all very simple and beautiful, but it is often the simple things, frequently overlooked, which are the most effective.

"So is the preparation made to heal, not an asthma, or duodenal, or a thrombosis, but to change a negative or uneasy state of mind to a positive or happy one, to banish the fear, to remove the anxiety or worry, to ease the nervous tension or irritability, to reassure the doubtful, to strengthen the exhausted, and give confidence to the over-diffident."

- Jane Evans,
"Introduction to the Benefits of the Bach Flower Remedies."

Whatever therapy you decide to try, remember that you are a unique individual; no-one can say what is best for *you*, but one thing that all patients need, in fact which is needed by everyone, is some tender, loving care. The human qualities of the practitioner, his or her ability to empathise with and spend time in really caring for the patient are of paramount importance, and may have a bearing on how successful the treatment is.

CHAPTER 14.
RELAXATION AND
BREATHING

In all diseases, whether it is rheumatoid arthritis, cancer, a virus infection or whatever, it is important to strengthen the immune system, so that we may be in an optimum a state of health and well-being as possible. The immune system is an incredibly complex system by which our bodies are able to resist disease and infection.

The most powerful tools we have to perform this task, to strengthen our resistance to illness are:-

1. The Mind/Spirit.

2. The food we eat.

3. The exercise we take.

4. Fresh air.

5. The rest we take, including sufficient sleep.

6. The ability to relax both body and mind.

Being relaxed in mind and body has a wonderfully beneficial effect on the immune system and should ideally be part of our everyday existence. In the pressures of modern living this is a problem for most people, so a conscious effort needs to be made to attain the time for oneself. However busy we are, it is important to the harmony of the body not to feel "rushed" while fulfilling our duties and tasks; this causes stress and tension to arise. Often we tend to do things too speedily for the natural pace of our bodies, and need consciously to "slow down."

The ideal condition of the body is to be in a state of balance and equilibrium. This allows the natural energy, the healing energy to circulate, causing us to feel that we are in a beautiful state of harmony, where everything just "flows" for us.

Some ways in which we can reach this desirable state include meditation, relaxation, deep-breathing exercises, the Alexander Technique, the use of visualisation, or the practising of arts such as Chi Kung, Tai Chi, or yoga.

Some people, including myself, find that a period of time spent in relaxation, combined with deep-breathing exercises is invaluable. But what is meant by the term "relaxation?" It probably means twenty different things to twenty different people.

RELAXATION

"Relaxation" should not be confused with "recreation". There is a difference; sometimes our recreations are not relaxing at all! Complete relaxation involves "letting go," not only of the body, the joints and muscles, but of the mind too, completely to become immobile. This wonderful state allows the mind and body and yes, the spirit too, to become completely re-energised so that when we are ready to resume our tasks, we feel much better, with renewed energy, power and enthusiasm!

The question arises: when should you practise your relaxation?

In arthritis a common feature is a feeling of tiredness, fatigue even. The right time to relax, then, is when your body tells you to, that is, before you become over-tired. This may be around mid-day, or perhaps after lunch. You may be in the middle of a job, preparing vegetables perhaps, or cleaning, when suddenly you notice how tired you are. The body is telling you to drop everything, (not literally!) and lie down. It is as well to listen to this inner voice, as, if we try to persevere beyond this point, our efficiency and our effectiveness decrease; certainly the body will suffer more later on.

When preparing to relax, you may like to unplug the telephone (or switch on the answerphone) to ensure peace and quiet. Choose somewhere to lie where you can be comfortable, maybe on a settee or bed, or some people prefer the floor.

Lie down carefully, as you should always treat your body with awareness; the way we do things is important. (In the Alexander Technique, one of the principles is that the process of *doing* is more important than the *end* product.) Make sure that you are not too hot or too cold; perhaps cover yourself with a blanket. Place a comfortable pillow or cushion underneath the head. Loosen any tight clothing.

Some people prefer to lie in a semi-supine position, that is, with the knees bent and the feet flat on the bed, fairly close to the body, and about a hip's width apart. This position is recommended by Alexander teachers, especially if you have a back problem, and is excellent whether you have arthritis or not, as it gives maximum rest to the spine. You may however prefer to lie with the legs flat and the feet splayed out. Place the hands on the abdomen, not touching each other, or in a relaxed position on either side of the body. Your head should be in a balanced, central position, turned neither to the left nor the right. Re-adjust any part of your body which does not feel comfortable.

This preparation may take a little time at first to find the way which is most comfortable for *you,* but in a very short while you will find that it will only take a few seconds to assume your most comfortable position for relaxing.

Now to start the relaxing process, which involves simply ...letting go. Let go of the muscles, the joints, every part of your body, even the internal parts. Feel yourself sinking into the bed, deeper and deeper...Tell yourself to just "let go." The process is helped by slow, deep breathing.

At first, if you are not used to relaxing in this way, you may find difficulty relaxing "in one go." One aid to relaxation which you may like to try is to first of all *tense* each part of the body in turn, then relax it. So begin with the feet; breathe in *slowly,* and at the same time tense the muscles of the feet, bending the toes. Hold for a few seconds, -perhaps to the count of five, then as you breathe out, relax the feet completely. Next, put your awareness into the legs...tighten the calf muscles as you breathe in, pressing the backs of the knees down onto the bed, hold... and gently breathe out. Follow this with each of the different body parts, working upwards, -thighs and hips, abdomen, spine, chest, shoulders, hands, arms, neck, not forgetting the face and head ... tensing and relaxing; at the same time breathing deeply and gently. When breathing in, surround yourself with a feeling of calmness, tranquillity and peace. When exhaling, breathe out any tension in your body, or any negative feelings, such as fear, resentment, worry, anxiety, pain or discomfort. You might like to imagine these feelings leaving your body, streaming out through the hands and feet. When you reach the head, press the neck into the bed, tightening the muscles...relax. Then screw up the muscles of the face, making a "prune," then gently let go... don't forget the jaw, as often people are so intent on relaxing that they find themselves with clenched teeth and tense jaw muscles!

Now just feel that you are in a state of complete relaxation; the breathing should be deep and gentle, and every time you exhale, feel yourself go more and more deeply into this relaxed state. When you reach this point of being totally relaxed, it is quite natural to fall asleep, even if only for a short while. Even if you do not, or if you find that the mind is still active, you may like just to listen to yourself breathing, following the breath...just breathing in the peace and calmness, filling yourself with healing tranquillity and harmony.

When you are ready to rejoin the world, perhaps after twenty minutes or so, make sure that all your movements are gentle and slow, at least at first. You may like to start by moving the fingers and toes, "wiggling" them a little, then stretching and relaxing the hands, arms, feet and legs... gradually waking up the body. Finally have a good stretch... think of the way a cat awakens after a nap, with slow, graceful stretching movements. Then roll over onto your side if you wish, sit up, and feel the change in your body as you begin to move. Try to maintain the feeling of peace, performing your tasks with awareness, for the rest of the day if possible!

To help with the relaxation, there are some excellent cassette tapes available for guidance, or playing soft music may be helpful. There are also books on the subject, or you may like to join a class. However you do it, you will be sure to enjoy the benefits of this wonderful therapy within a short time, if not immediately. The importance of relaxation cannot be overestimated. It is impossible to be in a state of stress and be relaxed at the same time, so if you are able to relax, the stress or tension just disappears, problems and worries fade into the background and we feel much more calm and positive about everything, more able to cope with difficult situations in our lives.

It may not always be possible, in a busy life, to be permanently in a state of equilibrium, in which we manage to balance the different aspects of our nature. We have a "doing" side, the "yang" or left-brained, male principle side of ourselves, which governs the actions and the practical side of us, and the "being" side, the "yin" of Chinese taoist philosophy, or feminine right-brained principle, which is concerned with the intuitive, passive, more mystical part of our nature. It is important to try to balance these two sides in order to be a whole, complete personality. We may need to look carefully at the different areas of our lives to see that we are not expending too much time and energy in one direction rather than another, such as moving from one busy activity to the next, to the detriment of taking time for sufficient rest and relaxation.

BREATHING

"Inhalation fills us with new, clean ki (energy), energising your entire system. Exhalation is the powerful and relaxing breath which allows us to relax and reach out to life."

-Elaine Liechti, "Shiatsu."

The breathing used in relaxation is of paramount importance. Deep, yogic breathing is one of the most valuable tools I have ever had the good fortune to learn, and I am profoundly and eternally grateful to my friends the wonderful yoga teachers the benefit of whose experience I have received. Its value is immeasurable, giving you an incredible feeling of lightness, balance and well-being. Once mastered, it becomes second nature to you, part of your life, playing its part in calming you when you are distressed or nervous, helping you to sleep when you are in discomfort or disturbed by problems, slowing you down when you feel "rushed", and in all ways beneficial.

It is said that 70% of body waste is released through correct exhalation, utilising the complete diaphragmatic breath. In addition, this way of breathing gives an internal massage to vital organs and integrates the autonomic nervous system, which controls the body/mind system.

When preparing to practise the breathing, find a comfortable chair and loosen any tight clothing. Be aware of *how* you sit; be relaxed, but make sure that the back is straight and the crown of the head is pulled upwards; you might imagine that there is a cord from the top of the head to the ceiling, pulling you straight. Place the hands on the abdomen, fingers not touching.

Now breathe slowly and deeply into the abdomen, feeling it expand as you do so. When you have taken a complete breath, hold it for a few seconds, then begin to exhale. As you do so, feel the abdomen contracting under your hands until all the breath is expired. Count five seconds before beginning to take the next breath. Check that you are still relaxed and peaceful, making sure that the facial muscles are relaxed. Repeat this exercise three or four times, concentrating on the breathing and relaxation.

Next, put your awareness into the chest, placing your hands on the rib-cage. This time, when you inhale, concentrate on filling the chest area, feeling the rib-cage expanding under your hands, opening up the chest area; fill completely. Once again, count slowly up to five before beginning to exhale. When all the breath is exhaled, count five as before. Repeat several times.

Then move the hands to the top of the chest, over the breast-bone. Repeat the breathing exercise, filling the tips of your lungs. Count five as before, then slowly exhale. Do this three or four times. The counting, in fact, can be used throughout the breathing exercise. When breathing in count five slowly, hold for five, exhale for five, then count five again while "empty". After a while you may find that you can increase the length of the count to six, seven or eight as long as it feels comfortable for you, but only do what feels "right" for you. There is a word of caution here. Do *not* hold your breath if you have high blood pressure or a heart complaint.

For a full, deep breath, the breathing exercises are combined into one. First of all make sure that you are still sitting in an erect position. Move your consciousness into the abdomen; begin to breathe in, watching it expand, then continue into the chest area...then to the top of the lungs, filling completely in one, continuous long breath. As before, hold to the count of five, or whatever feels comfortable for you, then slowly begin to exhale, first allowing the chest to contract...then the abdomen...until you feel that all the air is expelled. Count as before.

When you have repeated the full breath about ten times, sit quite still for a few minutes. Be aware of all the sensations in your body...feel the peace. Listen to any sounds there are in the room or outside...let them go. Just relax and be happy...let your heart smile!

You can practise the breathing any time, wherever you happen to be, then after a while it becomes second nature to you; you find that you are doing it almost *all* the time, but of course, not usually breathing as deeply as in the foregoing exercise.

When practised in the fresh air, the benefits of deep breathing are enhanced enormously, especially while walking, and there is nothing more delightful than to be able to walk in the countryside, perhaps among some trees, breathing deeply their life-enhancing properties. Whereas we breathe in oxygen and exhale carbon dioxide, the trees take in carbon dioxide and exude oxygen, which is a tremendous arrangement for both them and us! When walking under trees the air always smells so clean, cool and fresh. The latin word "spira" means "air", but it also means "spirit." As Arnold Ehret says, "The 'breath of God' is in fact, good fresh air!"

Physical and breathing exercises, especially when done in the fresh air or near an open window, develop vitality and health. The breathing, plus relaxation, practised regularly, will also help to develop a calm, balanced outlook, and contribute greatly to the healing process.

"The greatest happiness is knowing that you are your own master; that nothing can overpower you; that you can accept whatever life has to throw at you without losing the balance of your mind. As equanimity arises, the other qualities of a pure mind unfold giving divine love for others, compassion for their feelings and joy in their successes."

- L.I.F.E. Foundation booklet,
"Shanti Prana Vipassana."

CHAPTER 15.
EXERCISE

"Maintaining a proper balance between rest and exercise and exercising properly are the keys to a successful arthritis exercise programme."

- The Arthritis Helpbook,
by Kate Lorig and James F. Fries.

Joints in arthritic and rheumatism patients should be regularly exercised, with a full range of movement, even when in pain. Regular exercise is important for the following reasons:-

1) It strengthens muscles and joints.

2) It increases the range of movement that you have.

3) It reduces pressure on compressed nerves.

4) It helps to prevent loss of calcium and therefore maintains strength of bone.

5) It increases stamina, and therefore reduces fatigue.

6) It prevents loss of function. "Use it or lose it."

Even if you have lost the use of a muscle or joint, you should persevere with the exercises; soon you should start to feel some improvement and see some results for your efforts.

Ideally you should exercise every day, but avoid exercising any hot, inflamed joints although they should be moved through the full range of motion, twice a day if possible. If you have over-exercised on one day it is best to take it easy the next day. You will discover your limitations as you go along. Again, listen to the "inner voice" of wisdom.

Arnold Ehret, in "Mucusless Diet Healing System", stresses that it is important to avoid extremes of any kind, whether exercising, bathing, eating or sleeping. Even too much joy and happiness can be harmful! As of course can extreme worry, hate or anger. In all things, moderation is the keynote.

Moderate but regular exercise enhances the immune system in that it has a beneficial effect on the mind, which in turn influences the immune system to work properly as it should. It also helps to prevent calcium loss from the bones, thereby discouraging osteoporosis, which often arises in older women.

An important part played by exercise is that it helps to lower anxiety and stress levels which contribute to physical illness. Unrelieved stress produces a hormone which suppresses the function of the immune system, so that anything which counteracts this, such as exercise, proves of enormous benefit. It should however be taken regularly to maximise the effects. Furthermore, regular exercise reduces patterns of habitual stress, which in turn prevents chronic disease from developing.

Because of the need to exercise on a regular basis, it is best to choose an exercise which you enjoy, so that you look forward to practising it!

When should you exercise?

It is best to take your exercise when you have the least pain and stiffness; when you are not tired; and when your medication (if any) is having the maximum effect. Warming-up exercises help to avoid injury and enable you to move with more flexibility. These include stretching exercises, or tapping the body all over to increase circulation. If you have poor mobility and/or considerable pain and stiffness it is easier to take your exercise after a warm bath or shower. The application of heat to affected limbs will also help, as also will massage, in preparation for exercise.

One excellent way of exercising regularly, which is enjoyed by increasing numbers of people, is performing yoga exercises. There is so much to yoga and it is not the place of this book to describe it in detail. Suffice it to quote that great yoga teacher, Indra Devi:-

"Yoga aims, first of all, at removing the very causes of ill-health which are brought about by insufficient oxygenation, poor nutrition, inadequate exercise and poor elimination of the body's waste products that poison the system. Secondly, through rhythmic breathing and concentration, as well as by influencing our glandular activity, Yoga can help to increase our mental capacities, sharpen our senses and widen our intellectual horizon. And finally, through meditation, it enables man to come closer to the realisation of his own spiritual nature."

- Indra Devi, "Yoga for You."

Yoga movements are performed very gently, and a great advantage is that you only do as much as your body feels able to do; there is no strain of any kind, and certainly no competition, not even with yourself! If you can join a group, so much the better, but if not, there are various books on the subject with exercises to follow at home. Video and cassette tapes are also available.

From my own point of view, all I can say is that I have found yoga to be of immense value over the years, as well as being extremely enjoyable. Sometimes I have gone to a yoga class feeling quite tired and "jaded," but have found that by the end of the session I am re-energised, with a feeling of equilibrium and renewed well-being.

Another wonderful way to combine exercise with breath is in the form of a beautiful oriental Art, Tai Chi. Like yoga, Tai Chi helps to release built up energy and stress. The movements are performed very slowly, with great awareness. Practising the complete form of Tai Chi co-ordinates mind, body, spirit and breath. It utilises balance, sensitivity, flexibility and "chi", - the life force or intrinsic energy which holds the material world together. Since it is performed slowly and gently, utilising the whole body/mind, Tai Chi is ideal for people suffering with arthritis.

More recently I have discovered Chi Kung. Literally translated, "Chi Kung" means "Stillness of Breath." In therapeutic Chi Kung specific breathing exercises are taught in conjunction with gentle exercises. These promote the flow of chi (Life Energy) within the body, which in turn activates the self-healing process.

Interestingly, the lady trainer of our class described how she had suffered with arthritis for twelve years before taking up Chi Kung. With continued practice she found that her condition improved dramatically, so much so that she decided to train so that she could teach it! She observed that meditation and diet also play a part in maintaining her state of health.

As for myself, the effects of the practice showed almost immediately. The joints and muscles felt easier, more flexible, pain started to diminish, and perhaps most exciting of all, when I do the exercises I feel energy vibrating through my body, which seems to have a powerful healing effect.

Exercises especially designed for rheumatoid arthritis patients are taught in hospitals, and tapes can usually be obtained from the physiotherapy or rheumatology department. My own tape has been in regular use since 1984. The exercises take about twenty-five minutes. When I omit them in the morning, due to an early appointment, then I try to fit them in later, perhaps in the evening. If two consecutive days are passed without exercising, I really notice the difference on the third day; the joints become more stiff and mobility decreases. So I have found it important to exercise each day if possible. Special care is needed if you have had joint replacements, as there are some exercises which you should not perform. A physiotherapist will give advice.

Apart from directed exercise, other forms of exercise are recommended. Gentle walking and swimming are excellent, also dancing if you are able! Even dancing by yourself is wonderful - playing some music and just moving gently round the room; swaying and bending the body and limbs is very relaxing. One particular form of dance which I greatly enjoy is the Gabrielle Roth type of dancing, called Five Rhythm Dancing, or "The Wave"; there is a video available of the same name. It is an extremely free and relaxed way of dancing, accompanied by a drum. I always feel better for this and the feeling of liberation is tremendous! The beneficial physical effects of this type of movement usually last throughout the following day.

Singing is a natural breathing exercise which is good for the lungs and chest area. I find that singing in the bath or shower is a particularly joyful thing to do, especially when you are feeling a bit "low." If you break into a song things suddenly look much more positive! I can highly recommend it.

Gentle gardening, if you can manage it, is wonderfully therapeutic, especially as it has the bonus of being in the fresh air. In fact, if you can perform *any* of your exercises outside, or by an open window, so much the better. Oxygen is a basic necessity to one's well-being.

Even if you are partially disabled, there are many varied exercises you could try. You may like to purchase a book describing exercises for arthritis patients, such as "The Arthritis Helpbook," (see Bibliography,) which, even apart from the exercises, is an excellent, comprehensive reference book for people with arthritis.

Whatever exercise you choose to do, make it your own, feel comfortable with it, and above all, enjoy it!

Michael A Weiner observes in his book "Maximum Immunity" that regular, vigorous, physical activity makes you feel alert and positive, and if you feel tense or depressed, your best remedy may be to get your body in motion!

CHAPTER 16
THE SPIRITUAL ASPECT

"And I have felt
A Presence which disturbs me with the joy
Of elevated thoughts; a sense of sublime
Of something far more deeply interfused,
Whose dwelling is the light of setting suns,
And the round ocean and the living air,
And the blue sky, and in the mind of man.
A motion and a spirit, that impels
All thinking things, all objects of all thought,
And rolls through all things."

- William Wordsworth, "Intimations of Immortality."

This book would not be complete without describing the help I have received on a "spiritual" level, and my growth and development in this direction, as this has had a bearing on the process of healing, at least in my case. The spiritual aspect has played, and continues to play, such an incredibly important and magical role in my life; however I shall endeavour to include here only those experiences which are relevant to the story, or connected with the process of healing, although I feel that the whole of it has had a profound effect on my ways of being, of thinking, indeed of the whole "me". To go further, I often feel that the "me" is no longer there; I am directed from somewhere else... I just have to flow with the Universal energy. To explain this a little more, I would say that the focus is more on the *feeling* part of me rather than the *thinking* (although of course I have to think as well!). This is graphically described in this quotation from a White Eagle book:-

"The way to truth is through the spirit. In the outer world is turmoil and unhappiness. You think with the mortal mind, with the mind which is part of the substance of earth. You should think with your inner mind; you should approach problems through the inner self, through intuition... You are looking outside for help, and all the time the help you want is inside. The world of spirit that so many of you talk about and believe in and long to touch, is all within."

- "The Quiet Mind," P.60.

This "Spirit" Presence has made itself more evident in my life in recent years. Ever since I was a teenager my conception of God has been that of a Great Spirit, a power of goodness and harmony, which can be found everywhere, in everything and everybody, if we look for it. This is a strong conviction, a "gut feeling", that satisfies my mind and my heart.

At certain times an overwhelming sense of beauty and harmony suffuses me with a wonderful sense of peace. One of these times is when making contact with the Earth - perhaps walking through the woods, or along a moorland pathway, or simply weeding the garden. Part of this harmony, I believe, comes through breathing fresh air, the life-giving energy, and feeling myself to be a part of Nature, of the vast tapestry of the Universe in its wondrous diversity. I suppose it is a traditional heritage of something ancient, mystical even, from times when we lived more closely to the earth than most people do nowadays.

"Set a time each day for quiet, perhaps wandering in the green places, the woods or country lanes; or, if this is not possible, by going into the green and sunlit countryside within your own heart. Seek the place of eternal silence, and in that silence you will receive your food - the bread and wine of life."

- White Eagle, from "Healing by the Spirit."

****

The synchronicity of how events "just happen" never ceases to amaze and delight me. There is an increasing belief that there is no such thing as coincidence. Right through life, you often find that one door opens the way to another. Looking back, you see that events were meant to happen in a certain order. You "happened" to be in a certain place at a certain time and something significant occurred, or you met someone who was a catalyst for change in your life in some way, even though you may not have realised it at the time.

In 1984 the contact with the "Great Spirit" began to make itself felt more strongly in my life.

As I previously described, when the arthritic symptoms became more evident, I was admitted into hospital for three weeks.

A friend, Eirlys, had given me a gift, a little book called "The Quiet Mind," from which I have quoted extensively in this chapter, as you may have already noticed! When I started to read the book, I was initially amazed at how appropriate were the messages on the page. It began to give me great comfort and inspiration when I most needed it. The magical thing thing about the book was that, when I was feeling really "low," perhaps in considerable pain, I would pick it up, hold it near my heart, "tune in" and open it at random. On the page where my eye alighted the relevant message would always be there, the perfect message for my situation or predicament at the time. Here is an example:-

After returning from hospital, one Saturday morning I awoke with severe pain, hardly able to rise out of bed, my spirits low. Reaching for the book, after "tuning in" I opened it and immediately read the following:-

"Do not despair; do not dwell on the negative side of any situation, for you will do no good by this. Always put into operation the forces of construction. Believe that good will come, that the best is coming, and it will. We shall never forsake you. We also are God's children and His agents. We shall never forsake you, dear brother."

- The Quiet Mind.

Can you wonder that I felt comforted? I felt that I had a direct line to some wonderful, compassionate Power. The first door had opened...

Then, in the following year, in the Spring, a friend of my husband's parents, a Polish lady, *happened* to mention that, from time to time, she attended a local healing group. I decided to go along one Sunday afternoon and to my surprise, discovered that it was a White Eagle Group! Immediately I connected this with my meaningful little book. Following this I became a regular attender at the Group meetings, held every fortnight. This proved to be a corridor which was to lead to the next waiting door!

The White Eagle Brotherhood is an undenominational spiritual organisation with a world-wide healing ministry, which began in the 1930's. At that time, a lady called Mrs. Grace Cooke started to receive and channel messages from a spirit being, who revealed himself as White Eagle, a Native American Indian in a past incarnation. Through these messages, which pointed the way to the source of all healing, the first White Eagle Lodge was opened in 1936, its purpose being "to heal... to comfort... to illumine..." Men and women go there to learn the the reason for their life on earth, and how to live and serve in harmony with the whole brotherhood of life, in health and happiness.

There are two main Lodges, one in Hampshire, the other in London. Healing groups are held in many towns and cities throughout the country. If you wish to know more about the work of the White Eagle Brotherhood there is an address to write to at the end of the book.

The White Eagle healers work on the subtle levels of the person, on the unseen bodies which surround our physical body, including the etheric and astral bodies, each with its own aura. Many people now believe that disease begins where there is an imbalance or disharmony in the subconscious mind, or subtle levels of a person. This lack of harmony over a period of time, leads to problems in the physical body, which are then the cause of illness or disease. If you wish to find out more on this subject there are many books available on Healing. One excellent one to start with is "Hands of Light," by Barbara Ann Brennan. (See Bibliography.)

With regard to contact healing, many people find much comfort in the physical contact, the experience of being touched by another person; this is especially important to people who have no partner, or who live alone and have little tactile contact with other people.

One definition of "Spiritual Healing" is the channelling of Universal energy to the receiver. The healer is merely an instrument for this energy, or life force, to flow through. The transference of energy is often a catalyst for the patient's own healing process to be set in motion - a "kick-start", you might say!

Ivan Cooke, the husband of Grace Cooke, was the author of a book called "Healing by the Spirit." In this he states,

"For most of us when we fall sick in body feel sick at heart...We want the healing touch deeply within ourselves - those infinitely tender and sensitive selves which we believe we successfully conceal from everyone, even from our own consciousness. What we long for, even unconsciously, is to be aware of the love of God."

- Healing by the Spirit.

At the White Eagle meetings I was certainly aware of a most beautiful and powerful Presence, and was privileged to receive healing from the kind and caring White Eagle ladies over a number of years. This must surely have had some bearing on my improvement!

What was this *Presence?* I did not know, but an event which happened early in the following year was to give me a tase of its wondrous love and wisdom.

Resentment is an emotion which is frequently found in people with arthritis. In 1985 I had an amazing, enlightening experience in connection with blaming others.

The fact was, I was partly blaming my husband for, as I saw it, contributing to the causes of my disease. For years I had felt that he had put his interests before me and the children. He had been building up a business and we hardly ever saw him, because in his spare time he was either playing football or golf. I ignored the fact that because he worked so hard he was in greater need of leisure pursuits. Anyway, I felt like a neglected wife! He never seemed to be there when I needed him most. So I was feeling rather sorry for myself, with a growing resentment.

One night in the spring of 1985, I was feeling worse than ever, lying in bed unable to sleep, wondering how I could spend the rest of my life with this person, when I had such negative feelings about him. I was near to despair, and in the darkness asked God for help.

Soon after this, lying there still unable to sleep, I "sensed" rather than heard a voice - which simply "spoke" three words inside my head:- "Saint Matthew Seven."

There was no mistaking the message, which had come into my head as clearly as if someone in the room had spoken. Straightaway I relaxed, repeated the three words to myself with a sense of curiosity, turned over and fell to sleep.

In the morning I fetched the Bible, turned to the New Testament, found Saint Matthew, Chapter Seven, and was astonished to discover the most beautiful, wise and profound words, words which were entirely appropriate for my attitude of mind:-

"Judge not, that you be not judged. For with the judgement you will pronounce you will be judged, and the measure you give will be the measure you get. Why do you see the speck that is in your brother's eye, but do not notice the log that is in your own eye? Or how can you say to your brother, 'Let me take the speck out of your eye', when there is a log in your own eye? You hypocrite, first take the log out of your own eye, and then you will see clearly to take the speck out of your brother's eye."

> \- The Bible, Revised Standard Version,
> St.Matthew Chapter 7.

To say I was astounded would be an understatement. Then I was struck by the wonderful grace I had received - a gentle and much-needed jolt, a lesson in compassion and humility. That I had been sent this lesson filled me with awe.

Another negative feeling is *fear*. Sometimes people are afraid of pain, illness, loneliness, old age and/or death.

White Eagle says:-

"If, by some miracle, fear of death could be removed, this in itself would go a long way towards healing all sickness. But this cannot come about until man begins to unfold his spiritual self, and then he attains a condition in which things formerly unintelligible begin to grow clear and luminous, and death becomes serene and beautiful, a mother come to succour man in his last deep need."

> \- White Eagle Calendar.

So, ideally, anything which troubles or disturbs the mind should be tackled and dealt with. Then, a positive, even joyful philosophy of life can enter in.

Disease often has the effect of bringing us back to the consciousness of God, and of His love for us. The more we experience of pain and problems, the greater the opportunity to become closer to God, to feel some sort of comforting Presence in our hour of need.

Ivan Cooke states,

"Truth must be realised in the heart. Book knowledge, intellectual pursuits will leave man ignorant of the deepest realities; only his own experience will teach him about God - these are the things which will lead man eventually to find God within his own breast."

- Healing by the Spirit.

In 1986, one of the White Eagle healers, Kay (who also happened to be my calligraphy teacher,) told me of a young man, a spiritual teacher, who was visiting Sheffield, giving talks and seminars. She asked me if I was interested in attending one of the meetings. I was busy all that week, right up to Friday. On that day I had a free evening, so I decided to go along - and that is how I first made contact with Dr. Patel, and the L.I.F.E. Foundation.

****

I have already described the incident in November 1988 when Dr. Patel gave a talk on the Nature and Causes of Disease, and the ensuing dynamic effects on myself and my life.

From that event, which instigated a great release of pent-up feelings, some of which had been suppressed for most of my life, I seemed to empty myself of negative feelings such as resentment and judgment, becoming more open to the power of the Spirit, with a new understanding of people and situations.

However there are always new lessons to be learned and challenges to be faced; these came frequently and were not always pleasant nor easy!

One of the lessons was presented to me in September 1990. I was angry with someone in the family. I made the mistake of having certain expectations which had not been fulfilled. I felt upset and disappointed, and extremely angry. If you have rheumatoid arthritis you will know that upset feelings cause physical pain; so it was in my case, so I decided to have a hot bath to ease the discomfort.

While in the bath I played one of Dr. Patel's cassettes of which the subject was "Attachment". Dr. Patel explained that attachment to feelings, people etc., can make us weak, causing us to blame other people and circumstances for our situation, when we need to depend more on ourselves. With a sudden surge of insight I realised that it all applied to me. Attachment implies that we depend on people, causing us to have expectations of them which are limiting to both them and to ourselves. The person I was angry with had no expectations of *me*, so I had to learn to have no expectations of *him*.

With regard to having feelings of disappointment and frustration, White Eagle says,

"Do not be discouraged. Learn not to be disappointed in anything, in any person. You are disappointed because your will, your desire, has been frustrated. Learn to submit to the Divine Will, for His Will is all-wise. Wait, then, for His appointments, learning to tread the path wisely, serenely."

- The Quiet Mind.

Another time, more recently, it was my daughter's birthday and I was preparing party food in the kitchen. But I wasn't enjoying myself very much. Indeed I felt rather annoyed as no-one was coming to help me and there was so much to do! So I asked the Universe for help. Suddenly, in a split second, everything was turned around. All the resentment vanished. I began to *enjoy* everything I was doing, and to prepare it all with great love and care, thinking of the enjoyment of the people who would consume it later.

One useful "dodge" to avoid being upset by "unfortunate" incidents which happen during the course of the day is something learned many years ago - how to change a negative happening into a positive one. I discovered that it was no use getting cross or upset about trivial incidents which are potentially annoying, if we allow them to be. An example of this is dropping things on the floor, which used to be a frequent occurrence with me as my hands are misshapen and often difficult. It doesn't happen so much nowadays; maybe I am learning the lesson! So if I spilt something on the floor I would determine that the floor would be cleaner after I had finished with it than it was previous to the incident. This immediately changed the situation and put me in charge of the whole business, with the challenge of making a clean floor, which would give me the satisfaction of seeing the results of my labours!

****

This chapter began by talking about flowing with the Universal energy, following the *still small voice* within and using my feeling part (intuition) rather than stilted intellectual thinking and planning. One of my greatest lessons was, and still is, always to listen to *that voice* which speaks within and knows just what my needs are.

At the beginning of this chapter I talked about listening to the body, or to the "voice of wisdom" and flowing with the Universal energy. One of my greatest lessons was, and sometimes still is, always to listen to that "still, small voice" within, that voice of intuition which knows just what I need to do, using my spontaneous feeling faculties rather than trying to plan everything.

"Understand that you yourselves must work in your everyday life; it is your reactions to daily events and to the conditions of life that really bring about attunement, achievement... The beginning of this work is your awareness of the still small voice within, of that gradually increasing Light in you which causes you to react as a gentle brother to all the conditions and all the circumstances of life."

- The Quiet Mind.

Everyone is capable of hearing his or her inner voice. If we sit in the stillness and silence this voice can be heard; with practice this becomes an increasing part of our lives, directing us not only in big issues but also in seemingly trivial matters.

What is this "voice?" I believe that it is the voice of intuition, our Higher Consciousness, the Divine Spirit, which is in all of us, whether we realise it or not. It can be recognised as such if it feels "right" to you; if it speaks with wisdom, truth and compassion. I have found that when I listen and follow its direction, things seem to go smoothly and well. When I disregard it, thinking "I" know better, then everything goes wrong. Projects become difficult, plans go askew, and all sorts of obstacles loom up!

****

For anyone with a physical problem, listening to the body is especially important. Nearly everyone has to spend time *unlearning* habits which have been instilled into us, usually from childhood, and which have become second nature to us, especially if and when we reach a stage of consciousness where we wish to understand and know ourselves better, so that eventually we can discover who we really *are*. First we have to unravel the knots of bad habits, such as tension, fear of speaking our true feelings, or not following our intentions with action, and so on. For me, one of the challenges is to relax when I need to. I tend to try fitting too many jobs into the time available during the day, often performing each task at a slightly faster pace than is natural to me, and therefore suffering from strain and even fatigue. Of course, this is counter-productive as I then have to take more rest. So I really have to listen to that voice when it says, "You are tired. Stop what you are doing and lie down *now*."

****

Learning consciously to slow down has been a valuable lesson in patience, which has never been one of my virtues! Patience really means trusting in the Universe that everything will work out all right; it means having faith. This is not always easy, as we often worry that things may not be conducive to our welfare, in that they may cause problems or discomfort.

Sometimes, before visiting a new venue or meeting place for the first time, I used to be a little apprehensive about certain things which may appear trivial - would there be a comfortable chair to sit on? Would the toilet be accessible? (i.e. on the same floor.) People with physical difficulties will understand these problems. But I have found that if it is "right" for me to go to a particular meeting - perhaps one connected with self-development, healing, the Environment and so on, then things are usually comfortable and available!

On the subject of patience, White Eagle declares:-

"Patience really means confidence in God, knowing that God has you in His care. God...is all around you and in you and is working out a wise and beautiful purpose in your soul. Do not live with the feeling that you must get over the ground as quickly as possible to reach a certain point. Just live every moment, every hour, every day, tranquilly in the protective love of God, taking the hours as they come and doing one thing at a time, quietly."

- The Quiet Mind.

It is my belief that the greatest achievements are not the visible, material ones, of jobs completed satisfactorily, although this has its merits of course, but the *inner* achievements, of making progress in conquering, our *selves,* to become more spiritually aware, loving, caring and compassionate beings, serene in the knowledge of our own nature.

Having faith in the Spirit, or the Universe, or whatever is your own personal belief, means that you surrender everything to this Power, so that you begin to flow, you just flow with whatever you happen to be doing. This brings a wonderful sense of tranquillity. When this happens, your tasks become easy - everything just falls into place.

"Only where there is trust can faith arise, and where there is faith there is freedom from fear and agitation; in the absence of fear and agitation one arrives at a point within oneself of deep contentment, deep respect and reverence for life."

- Dr. Patel.

How can we achieve this?

I have already mentioned affirmations in another chapter. There is no doubt that their usefulness in reprogramming the mind is quite extraordinary. You would have to practise them to believe their value. Furthermore, through them you can help to bring to yourself whatever qualities you wish, whether it be trust, faith, patience or whatever.

What has all this to do with healing? you may ask. The answer is, once again, that your state of well-being is dependant to an enormous degree on how you are integrated as a person, that is, how you are at-one with yourself in all areas of your being, which includes your mind and spirit, as well as your body.

Sometimes it is especially difficult to keep calm and tranquil in all circumstances, for example if you are experiencing a great deal of pain, or perhaps someone has hurt or annoyed you in some way, or for some other reason. I have found that one way to "get back to myself", to restore equanimity, is to meditate.

The mention of meditation is daunting to some people. But meditation does not necessarily mean going into a separate room and sitting in the silence for hours each day. It means simply being aware of your own presence, and the existence of a Greater Presence inside yourself; it means feeling the power and truth of the Spirit.

"How many people have ever discovered the power of their own presence? To do nothing, to say nothing....just by the power of one's own presence the mind begins to unfold just as a flower blossoms."

- Dr. Patel.

If you can set aside some time for prayer and meditation, perhaps first thing in the morning, (even if it means getting up earlier!) you find that after a while this time becomes increasingly precious and meaningful to you. In fact for many people it becomes the most important time of the day. I have found that the busier I am, or the more problems I have, the greater the importance of "doing my practice."

It is wonderful on a dull, dark morning to sit with a lighted candle, in the stillness and silence, or even on *any* morning. With practice, you begin to feel other Presences with you in the room. I do not wish to discuss what happens during meditation in too much detail, as each person's esoteric experience is personal, private... and even sacred. Suffice it to say that wonderful insights, intuitions and realisations often come during this time, and frequently the feeling that you are being guided... It is my belief that we all have a Guardian or Companion Angel, whose sole (soul!) task it is to help and guide us on our journey through life. Some people think of this as the Higher Self.

With regard to angels, White Eagle has this to say:-

"When you meditate, remember the angels. Call upon them, breathe in their love, their wisdom, their power.

Meditate on the angels of the earth, of the air, of the fire and of the water. Try to attune yourself to these angelic powers and receive from them the light and power and the life that you need in your service to the world."

-White Eagle Calendar.

When we ask our angels for help we start to feel that we are not alone - our angels are co-operating with us to fulfil our duties and concerns, whether they be enormous undertakings or the ordinary small tasks of every day. We start to feel that there is help and guidance all around us. I should add that this only seems to work when our work is of an unselfish nature, when our motives are of the highest. If we ask for something for ourselves which is not an essential need, it is quite likely not to work! However, the power of prayer is incredible, having an amazing, positive effect not only on the people we pray for, but also on ourselves. The growing power brought to us through meditation and prayer produces unimaginable effects, among other things increasing our moral and emotional strength, courage, hope, self-esteem and self reliance.

As the trust in our abilities and capabilities increases we find a growing strength and courage of conviction, so that we discover it becomes easier to make decisions; we just feel, and often even *know,* the right course to take. The magical outcome of this is that we begin to rely upon our own resources, taking personal responsibility for all our activities, our body, health and the way we live. And taking personal responsibility for ourselves is really the only way to live a successful and happy life, really using our potential and our talents to fulfil ourselves as individuals. We become intensely aware of our surroundings and the events which occur in our lives, so that we begin to savour each moment and live every experience to the full, not thinking too much about the past or the future, so that we stop worrying or even making too many plans.

When this happens, we immediately start to see everything in a different light. We stop blaming others, judging and/or criticising. We become more decisive and self-assured, more willing to attempt activities without waiting for others to take the initiative. We become more tolerant and understanding of other people's problems.

Other results of meditation include the development of the intuition, greater clarity of vision, and increasing awareness, in all kinds of ways.

Becoming more aware predisposes a greater consciousness towards people around us, to our environment, and to the Earth which nourishes and sustains us. In fact we begin to sense a feeling of unity and harmony with all things, all creatures and the Earth itself - that everything is interconnected.

****

It is only during the twentieth century that physicists in the Western world have made remarkable discoveries which have turned traditional physics on its head. These discoveries, in atomic physics, are concerned with the nature of matter; with the substances from which everything is formed, every leaf, rock, all creatures, fossil fuels - in fact, every single thing on this planet, including you and I!

For hundreds of years physicists have been trying to fathom out the fundamental laws which govern natural phenomena, but it only been during the last ninety years, with the use of modern instruments, that dynamic experiments were able to be performed, which have enabled scientists to obtain glimpses of the essential nature of things.

Kathryn Lausevic

These experiments have produced exciting and revolutionary results.

Instead of the elements and substances being separate and different from one another, the scientists have found that everything is interconnected. It is the interaction between electrons and atomic nuclei which form the basis of all matter:-solids, liquids, gases, living organisms and all biological processes. To put it more simply, after studying the atom it was discovered that all substances are made up of atoms; the sort of substance it is, is determined by the number of electrons, protons and neutrons contained in its nucleus. Everything is mutable; matter is energy and all particles can be transmuted into other particles. The whole Universe becomes a beautiful web of interconnected patterns. A particle cannot be seen in isolation, but is an integrated part of the inseparable whole. The Universe is the body of God, if you like, and each of us is a cell in God's body. What a beautiful and incredible discovery!

Particles flow and change into other particles, so the integral principle of all things seems to be movement, flow and change. Of course, *all* life is included in this - meaning every human being. I believe that this means that movement, flow and change are an integral part of each one of us. Problems arise when we do not "flow" with life, when we become static, either physically - not sufficiently exercising our bodies, or mentally, becoming rigid in our thinking, not being open to new ideas or being willing to listen to others' opinions, or even emotionally, living in the past, retaining old outworn feelings of resentment, anger, sadness, fear or other negative feelings which hinder us from being able to express our true selves.

We need to be willing to change ourselves according to what is needed for our growth; to flow with life and to be flexible to whatever arises in our day-to-day activities. I have discovered that if I am willing to change according to what is needed at a particular moment, perhaps doing something completely *different* from the *usual,* I start to feel some sort of "magic" and harmony working and life becomes an exciting adventure!

The knowledge, that we are interdependent with everything and interconnected with one another, gives us a different perspective on the way we see things. Instead of feeling that we have to conquer and tame nature, to "lick" it into the shape *we* want, we have a sense of wishing to co-operate with it, to live in harmony with it, and with all of life including all living things. We are merely a part of a greater integrated, self-regulating organism. Furthermore, we can identify with each person; all people are our brothers and sisters. We are all cells in the body of God. In that case, whatever we do to others we do to ourselves.

When we feel this unity, this unconditional love, it initiates a desire in us to share things with others, to help those less fortunate than ourselves, especially when we are so privileged; we in the west have so much in the way of material comforts compared with the greater part of the world's population; how can we ignore the plight of the starving, the homeless, the animals used in laboratory experiments, or indeed, the environmental state of the earth, our communal home of which we are the stewards. We feel an obligation to do our best to help redress the balance, if we are able.

Nowadays more and more people are becoming aware of the plight of the planet. Many of them share a strong sense of wishing to serve in some way, knowing that the time is short before the crucial point of no return. This consciousness is now accelerating throughout the whole world, in some countries at a tremendous rate. Little pockets of "aware" people and groups are springing up all over the place

- planetary consciousness is spreading at a rate of knots! There is a theory which claims that when a certain percentage of people reach a high level of consciousness, then *everyone* will also achieve that level. This is called Morphic Resonance, or Hundredth Monkeying, and it is evolution in our lifetime. This has been seen demonstrated in animals which learn new habits, and also applies to human beings. The babies of the next generation are born with the blue print of the new pattern. This is why the babies nowadays seem so alert, so bright and intelligent. It is all very exciting.

****

"Be thankful for every opportunity to serve which is laid before you."

- The Quiet Mind.

When you are helping someone your attention is completely focused on that person. The spin-off from this is that you completely forget yourself and your own problems. But of course this is not the ideal motive for serving.

Spiritually awakened people serve because they cannot help it. They see what needs doing and they do it. The best way I can describe it is a feeling of being a "channel" for God's work, surrendering oneself to the will of the Divine. It is part of the flowing. Furthermore it has a healing effect, as the energy flows through us. Paul Lambillion, Healer, Counsellor and Spiritual teacher, in a magazine article observed that by developing a willingness to serve, we empower the love in us so that it can flow freely and do its work as it knows best. He also declared that through love, we give freedom, not in binding but in liberating all whom we meet along the way.

Service can take many forms; helping family and friends; serving the community; animal welfare... there are so many causes and people who need our help. And giving the help has the effect of making us feel we have worth, bringing wholeness, peace and even joy.

"Whatever we give spirals out into the Universe - and beyond! Like throwing a pebble into a lake, the ripples extend out endlessly. Every single act of friendship creates a powerful thought process that echoes around the whole world, even of it is only making someone a cup of tea, or massaging their shoulders when they are tired."

- Dr. Patel.

The magical thing about giving is that you discover that the more you give, whether it is of service or anything else, the more you receive. You find that all sorts of wonderful things come back to you, not necessarily in material benefits, but to the spirit within, creating a beautiful feeling of grace, well-being and happiness.

The feeling of grace also arises when you feel and express gratitude, whether you are thanking a friend for their help with a problem, or remembering to thank your nearest and dearest for the small, helpful tasks they do each day. Equally important, if not more so, is giving thanks to God.

"The light that shines from a thankful heart can illumine the whole of life, and if you give thanks each day to God you will be surprised how much more smoothly and easily the wheels of life will run."

- Healing by the Spirit.

There is so much to be thankful for; numerous small delights, the perfume of a flower, the sun shining through trees, the sound of a friend's voice; all the things which lighten our hearts. We also need to thank God for our challenges, for our problems! It is often through the challenges that wonderful perceptions and realisations come to us, because wrapped up in each problem is the gift of a lesson, if only we look for it - a special gift meant just for us, to take to heart, assimilate, and remember. The Universe provides us with the appropriate opportunities for our development. *We are in exactly the right place at the right time*, and if we keep coming up against the same situation, or if the same problem keeps recurring maybe it is because we have not sorted it out properly yet - there is still something to be learned from it. It may be patience, trust or some other quality which we need for our growth.

If you are in a relationship you will know that this can cause all kinds of "problems". But it is from these that we have the opportunity to learn the most important and precious lessons - such things as tolerance, keeping serene when small "annoyances" arise, or accepting that other people's opinions are as valid as our own, and so forth. If everyone "got on" harmoniously, what would we learn? By definition, just being here on the Earth implies that we have difficulties to overcome, to further our development. The greater the difficulty, the greater the victory when we master it. So, if you have many problems to face, feel privileged! You have an opportunity for gentle growth and development.

"A time of crisis is a time of great opportunity."

-Chinese proverb.

Most of us are looking for help and inspiration, especially if we are experiencing pain, whether physical or emotional. A secure faith is a source of continuous support and regeneration. All the great Masters and teachers inspire us with their words of wisdom, truth and compassion, and for myself it has been a great privilege to receive the benefit of the teachings and knowledge of some enlightened beings, including some people whose workshops I have attended and books I have read, to all of whom I owe unlimited gratitude and send much love.

Although we can choose to take the teachings of the Great Masters on board, ultimately we come back to ourselves. We can find that power within ourselves, joyfully following our own truth which leads towards integration of body, mind, emotions and spirit.

So what does it all boil down to? I believe that the basis of it all is LOVE. If you live your life with love and compassion, that is all that matters; it is not necessary to belong to an "accepted" religion, or think of yourself as religious.

I would like to finish this chapter with a quotation which seems so simple as to be obvious; nevertheless it is a profound Universal truth, which I think is appropriate for our present planetary crisis:-

"Love alone can save the world."

PART 3.
SOME THEORIES
ON THE CAUSES OF
RHEUMATOID ARTHRITIS

CHAPTER 17
HYPOTHETICAL CAUSES

"Any science or health-care system based on the physical world is based on secondary causes, not primary ones."

- Barbara Ann Brennan, "Light Emerging."

When I first wrote this chapter it appeared as a set of disconnected facts, a jumble of information with no link between the separate parts, rather like an orchestra playing different tunes at the same time.

Since then, in fact very recently I have discovered some exciting information which puts the whole subject of the causes of rheumatoid arthritis into a new perspective - could it be the missing piece of the jigsaw? I have a strong sense that it may well be; at least I hope it will contribute something to the whole picture. Furthermore it seems to allow everything to fall into place. You could say that one thing leads to another...

The word "dis-ease" speaks for itself. Anything which is contrary to the harmony of our being, causing us not to be at ease with ourselves, especially over a considerable period of time, and which is not dealt with, can lead to illness on a physical level. This seems to be true of rheumatoid arthritis.

The causes of R.A. are complex and sometimes deep-rooted. I believe the way the disease manifests in the body is not a simple process. Although the causes are almost certainly connected, for the sake of clarity I shall put them into different categories, as there are the "unseen" causes, connected with the mind, emotions, personality and so on; then there are the precipitating causes which can trigger the disease (these too may not be apparent). Finally there are the physical factors, the processes by which the disease develops in the body.

Although the causes of the condition are diverse in one sense, you will see as the chapter unfolds that there is a common thread, a link between each of the various symptoms and conditions. The basic reason for the disease to manifest may be a different one for each person; maybe from experiences from our past, perhaps dating back to childhood, or even from previous lives, if you believe in that. Whatever the individual reason for one's illness, what these causes have in common is that they are mainly connected with *stress* of one sort or another.

I have no medical background so please bear with me as I attempt to describe these hypotheses.

HOW IT BEGINS

Many health-care professionals nowadays realise that disease begins on subtle levels, in the "unseen" energy field that surrounds the body. This happens before it manifests in the physical body.

Barbara Ann Brennan, in her book "Light Emerging," claims that we create our own experiences. This includes whether we experience health or disease. All our creativity rises from our deeper selves, the essence of who we are, which is our basic reality. Health is a result of expressing our true essence through our consciousness, mind, feelings and our physical body. You could say we are being "true to ourselves."

Dis-ease occurs when we block the expression of our deeper selves from coming through all levels into the physical. This can happen on an individual basis, but also certain diseases tend to occur in different cultures, for instance, there may be a greater incidence of heart disease, a stress- and diet-related disease, in a culture where living is stressful and not too much attention is paid to nutrition.

In disease, we have separated ourselves from our true, unique selves.

This idea, that blocking one's creative power is a factor in rheumatoid arthritis was demonstrated by research carried out by George Solomon, a doctor who made an extensive study of the emotional and personality factors in the onset and course of autoimmune disease, particularly rheumatoid arthritis. In 1981 Dr. Solomon published his findings, in which he stated that the arthritic process was *always* the expression of a personal conflict.

There seem to be specific personality traits connected with different conditions or diseases. Rheumatoid arthritis has been studied extensively over the years to try to discover the underlying causes of the disease. From this, a basic personality type has emerged.

In describing the R.A. personality, Dr. Solomon found that rheumatoid arthritics were extremely dependant, felt inadequate, had difficulty coping with their environment and with other people, and were *severely blocked in emotional expression.* They frequently denied their dependancy by over-compensating with an outward facade of independance, self-assurance, and self-control. Arthritic people tend to turn their anger inwards rather than expressing it.

Solomon set up a study to compare women arthritics with their non-arthritic sisters. The arthritic women described themselves as "moody, highly strung, nervous, tense, and easily upset." They were perfectionists and sensitive to criticism and perceived "rejection;" that is, they felt rejected if anyone slighted or criticised them, or even if they *thought* they had been criticised, even though it may have been misconstrued. They found it difficult to express their feelings, especially of anger with their spouses and children. Almost every arthritic patient could trace the onset of the disease to an acute or chronic stress situation. So state of mind is a crucial factor.

Among children with r.a. there was a high incidence of youngsters whose parents were divorced, separated or widowed. Adoption was three times more common among the arthritic children than among a comparative control group. Within a short time the onset of the disease occurred in about half of the children who had experienced traumatic events.

In the book, "Love your Disease," John Harrison, a doctor and practitioner of complementary medicine puts forward the hypothesis that we *choose* to be ill, because this condition protects us against aspects of our personality which frighten us and which we would prefer to ignore. So we choose to be ill rather than deal with the deeper issues. By the same token, once we understand the reasons for our illness, by being receptive and open we can begin the healing process. The unresolved issues, he declares, usually date from events in childhood which form the basis of our behaviour, our thinking and expectations. This means that even our responses to recent events are already mapped out, as we have acquired certain thought patterns.

A person who feels "controlled" by external events is more likely to be ill than one who feels the freedom of being in charge of his/her life, who claims the power of choice in organising how they want their life to be.

Dr. Harrison puts forward the idea that a person suffering from a mobility-related disease such as arthritis may have a fear of being fully mobile because of the demands and responsibilities that full mobility might impose. For some women it is sometimes a way (albeit unconsciously) of getting some loving care from an insensitive or undemonstrative husband!

Men with arthritis are often angry. They may have feelings of frustration and/or dissatisfaction, or of being unloved, which cause deep-seated sadness, but in our society being sad is not so acceptable in a man, so he will choose to be angry.

All negative emotions affect us, causing the sort of stress which leads to physiological changes in the body, connected with the immune system, and rheumatoid arthritis is thought to be an immune-related disease.

THE IMMUNE SYSTEM.

The immune system has two main functions:-

1. To arrange for unwanted cells to be destroyed.
2. To encourage healthy cells to protect the body.

The primary organ of the immune system is the thymus gland. There are some cells called "T-cells" which are thymus related; these cells help to keep the body in balance. If they are impaired, disease can manifest.

Why should this happen?

The primary cause of T-cell depletion is **free oxidising radicals.** (Described in Chapter 11.) Free radicals cause destruction of the joints.

Stress plays an enormous part in depressing the immune system. Suppression of emotions - fear, anxiety, anger, in fact stress of any kind leads to the release of a certain hormone, adrenalin, which has an adverse effect on the immune system. (The adrenal glands are also stimulated by sugar, caffeine and nicotine.)

Of course, a certain amount of stress is a normal part of everyday living; but we are talking here about *unrelieved* stress, such as long-term suppressed emotion.

Dr. John Harrison declares that there is a connection between the *suppression of anger* and *liver dysfunction.* The liver processes everything we eat and if the liver is not functioning properly then our food is improperly digested. This in turn leads to a build up of waste material and toxins in the intestines and the colon. (More about this later.)

Additional factors which weaken the Immune System:-

Ageing, which causes shrinking and hormone depletion.

The use of steroids and other drugs.

Toxins.

Smoking.

Taking antibiotics, especially over long periods.

Nutrient deficiencies, such as protein, vitamin and mineral deficiencies, and lack of essential fatty acids. Saturated fats contained in meat can cause inflammation. Intake of sugar, including fruit sugar and honey. (The effects of sugar last five hours.)

Removal of organs. e.g. tonsils, appendix, gall bladder. (I have had all of these removed!)

Lack of sleep. Sleep regulates the immune system. People under the least stress need less sleep.

Some Precipitating Causes of Arthritis

A traumatic event can trigger the onset of the disease, such as a bereavement, the loss of a close relationship or a sudden shock.

In a person who is holding onto tension and stress in the mind or body, the disease could start at any time, often in later life, if the problem has not been addressed.

Other possible "triggers" include:- *allergy, infection, toxins,* or, as already mentioned, an excess of free oxidising radicals.

PHYSICAL CONTRIBUTORY FACTORS IN RHEUMATOID ARTHRITIS

Toxins

Nowadays, we are all exposed to toxins from food, drugs and the environment. The combined effect of chemical toxins is thousands of times greater than the sum of the effects of the individual chemicals. No-one can say what are the effects of the thousands of toxins we are exposed to. Apart from these chemicals with which we all come in contact, such activities as smoking, drinking alcohol to excess or taking drugs are some of the main reasons for an accumulation of toxins in the body.

In his book, "Detoxification and Healing", Dr. Sidney MacDonald Baker states that detoxification is the most important activity in the body's function. This process, getting rid of toxins, can take place in the wall of the intestine, in the lungs, or the toxins can pass into the blood supply to be detoxified by the liver.

From a liver test carried out at Great Smokies Diagnostic Laboratory (address at end of book), the result showed that I was a "pathological detoxifier", i.e. the amount of toxins was greater than the liver could deal with, causing imbalances. It looked as though I was a heavy smoker, took drugs or was a chronic alcoholic. But I never smoke, have not taken any drugs for years, and cannot remember when I last had an alcoholic drink! So how and why did I have so many toxins in my body?

I had purchased a cassette tape from I.O.N., called "Rejuvenation with Phytonutrition," by Dr. Jeffrey Bland. At the end of Dr. Bland's lecture, someone asked a question which made me sit up. It was to this effect:-

In a pathological detoxifier who does not smoke, drink or take drugs, where do the toxins come from?

Dr. Bland's answer was that in a pathological detoxifier, where the toxins do not come from external sources such as those mentioned, then they must be produced **inside** the body, from an excess of BACTERIA.

This rang bells in my mind, as it was not the first time I had heard of this idea. It seemed to be targeting me from diverse and unexpected sources.

BACTERIA, PARASITES AND YEAST OVERGROWTH

Of course we all house bacteria, or germs in the gut, to perform all kinds of tasks, in digestion, etc. Most bacteria are harmless. But there are also "pathogenic" bacteria, which take nourishment from us without giving anything in return. In fact they actually harm our bodies.

As bacteria and also any parasites which may be in the intestines consume our food, they produce waste products - new chemicals which overload the main detoxification system, which is contained in the liver. An overburden of toxins, with not enough support for the liver, causes problems of imbalances and liver dysfunction.

If this condition is accompanied by an overpermeable mucosa, i.e. "leaky gut" (see below), the undesirable waste matter passes from the intestine into the bloodstream, to be circulated round the body, causing inflammation and pain in muscles and joints. It can also cause allergies or food intolerances.

My way of dealing with the resulting discomfort was to detoxify more. This caused a depletion in the reserve of sulphur, the main element in detoxification, therefore furthering the liver's inability to detoxify. So it was a vicious circle!

When this happens, any dietary or environmental insult can trigger more inflammation.

When our food is metabolised a process called "burning" occurs. During this process bacteria produce "smoke" which is normally passed out through the bowel, but some of it is absorbed into the body, and then has to be detoxified and excreted. Research is still continuing as to how harmful these substances are.

Toxins can also be produced in the upper intestinal tract, when bacteria get hold of a vitamin or mineral with which they have a particular affinity. The toxins they produce again provoke all kinds of symptoms, depending on the person.

We are all giving house-room to unwanted "guests" whether we realise it or not. These include anything that lives on or in our bodies:- bacteria of course, (although many are beneficial,) worms of all kinds, fungi, viruses, moulds and mites. These are influencing our health to various degrees.

By many authorities parasites are now considered to be the cause of symptoms and illness, although they are also found in people who have *no* symptoms. One British researcher, Dr. Roger Wynburn-Mason, suggests that a parasite, Endolimax nana, is the cause of rheumatoid arthritis as well as a whole host of collagen-related diseases. This parasite, E. nana, is transmitted through tap water and contaminated food. Some researchers believe that even if this particular parasite is not responsible for rheumatoid arthritis, there is some kind of organism which *does* cause it, in susceptible individuals. Dr. Wynburn-Mason's book is called,"The Causation of Rheumatoid Disease and Many Human Cancers: A New Concept in Medicine." (Please see Bibliography.) Unfortunately it is not available in the U.K.

Signs of parasitic infection in adults include **arthritis**, autoimmune disease, food allergy, bowel disorders, fatigue, diarrhoea, flatulence, gastritis, headaches and numerous other symptoms.

Having had a recent test for parasites, on receiving the result I was interested to find that I *did* have a parasite. The one which is inhabiting my body is called BLASTOCYSTIS HOMINIS. This parasite was once thought to be commensal (harmless), but is now considered to be a pathogen (i.e. one which causes symptoms and illness). In many people there are no symptoms; in others, however, this parasite can cause symptoms such as irritable bowel, chronic fatigue, and **arthritic and rheumatic complaints.**

So what causes the body to be inhabited by unwanted bacteria and/or the presence of parasites?

The answer is, a **weakened immune system**. (The reasons for this have already been described.)

A lowered immune system increases the risk of infection by these undesirable organisms. It is rather like a houseplant which has become unhealthy and is infested with flies and other insects.

Please see Chapter 18 for more information on parasites and how to deal with them.

On television I was spellbound by a programme which described a condition called "Autobrewery Syndrome". I realised it applied to me. (Please also see Appendix 2 - Candida.)

This condition occurs when sugar or yeast ferments to alcohol in the body.

Sugar, the common source of energy for all living things, releases energy by "burning", producing pure water, pure carbon dioxide and energy. However, it can burn incompletely, breaking down into pieces which contain units of two or three components which make up the sugar. The two-unit product is alcohol. Everyone makes about half an ounce of alcohol per day in the intestines, which is taken into the system. The alcohol is toxic as it interferes with the enzymes of the body chemistry. It is normally detoxified by the process of burning.

If the body chemistry has been unbalanced by intestinal surgery or, more commonly, by *antibiotics,* which indiscriminately kill "good" as well as "bad" bacteria in the gut, there is often a proliferation of yeast germs, which consume sugar and convert it into alcohol in the intestinal tract.

The alcohol has a particularly destructive effect on one of the groups of enzymes which are the main workers in the detoxification system of the body. The alcohol takes over, becoming a sort of master toxin, enhancing the toxicity of all the other toxic substances. Furthermore it interferes with the activity of the key enzymes which transform fatty acids into hormones.

OVERPERMEABLE GUT ("LEAKY GUT") AND FOOD INTOLERANCES

The wall of the gut is permeable, to some extent, to allow certain substances, such as key nutrients, to pass through. Sometimes, however, this boundary between the intestinal tract and the rest of the circulation breaks down, which then allows undesirable matter to pass through into the bloodstream. This prompts the immune system to deal with the "intruders", causing a reaction in the joints. This in turn causes inflammation.

What are the causes of gut overpermeability?

a   Food allergies and intolerances, which weaken the wall of the digestive tract. Allergens can be tested by a simple blood test. (See Chapter 6 - Testing for Food Allergies.) Food intolerances or sensitivities are very common in people with arthritis.

I realise that I have stated that "leaky gut" can be both the cause of, and the result of food allergies. It appears to be a vicious circle. One thing can exacerbate the other, and each condition allows for the other to happen. As Steven Terrass of Solgar succinctly remarked recently, "No leaky gut - no food allergies."

b) An excess of oxidants as opposed to antioxidants. Oxidants help the body to fight intruders, but can also initiate inflammation. If there are too many oxidants in proportion to the antioxidants, the mitochondria - the body's energy factories - suffer damage. The liver too, produces oxidants if overburdened with toxins.

One of the oxidants linked with arthritis (and also asthma and migraine) is nitric oxide. Levels can rise after ingesting allergens or breathing in toxins, such as smoke-filled or polluted air. Fried food is also a trigger. As well as causing inflammation there can be damage to the gut and lungs.

c) Candida albicans. The "fungus" state of candida, produces "antennae", which can penetrate the wall of the mucosa. (See Appendix 2 - Candida.) The result of this is that many substances are able to pass into the bloodstream, causing a wide variety of food and environmental allergies.

Other contributory factors to food sensitivities include:-

i. a weakened immune system;

ii. a lack of digestive enzymes - 90% of people with chemical sensitivity produce inadequate amounts of digestive enzymes;

iii. frequent exposure to foods containing irritants such as gluten in wheat (this can be a cause of "leaky gut");

iv. faulty nutrition, which can cause imbalances in the intestinal flora (micro-organisms). This again can trigger candidiasis.

These problems cause gut dysbiosis which in turn leads to inflammation.

In "leaky gut" condition, or if the digestion is incomplete, peptides (small sections of amino acids) can enter the bloodstream. Recent research has shown that peptides from gluten (found in grains) and casein (found in mammals' milk) are especially suspect in causing problems in susceptible individuals.

Furthermore, improperly digested proteins form large protein molecules which are toxic. Some form histamine which causes gastric secretion and is connected with acid build-up, which leads to pain and stiffness. A healthy liver can process histamine in the normal way but a damaged one has difficulty dealing with it.

Histamine is contained in certain amino acids and is a normal constituent of fermented foods, such as cheese and sauerkraut, although amounts are usually small. It is also found in fermented drinks such as wine and beer, sausage, tomato, spinach, yeast extracts, bananas and avocados. Histamine levels rise dramatically in certain foods during storage, such as stored fish, due to bacterial activity.

Histamine is released in the body during allergic or inflammatory reactions. Sometimes too much is produced and causes strong reactions. It is often difficult to distinguish between reactions to histamine and reactions to allergens or other food intolerances, because the effects of histamine mimic symptoms to true allergens. Together with other mediators, such as tyramine, they produce symptoms of an allergic reaction which attempts to rid the body of an invading allergen.

The effects of histamine may be increased in people who are taking certain drugs, which interfere with enzyme activity.

OTHER POSSIBLE CONTRIBUTORY FACTORS IN RHEUMATOID ARTHRITIS

1) **"Constipation.** -One of the most common "illnesses" of the western world.

When a person is constipated toxins and waste material are retained in the body. Sometimes the person may not realise they are constipated, as they pass regular motions, but there may be caked-on material in the colon which has accumulated over years, very often since childhood. These waste acids can enter the bloodstream, causing stiffness and pain as they are circulated round the body.

2) **A weak ileo-caecal valve.**

If the valve between the small intestine and the colon has become weakened, faecal matter can leak back from the colon into the small intestine. This may include bacteria which should not be present in the small intestine. This waste matter and bacteria can then be absorbed into the bloodstream, to be circulated round the body, causing stiffness and pain.

3) **Hormonal imbalances.**

Thyroid imbalances, which underlie blood sugar imbalances and oestrogen imbalances (especially in women after the menopause) can cause loss of calcium. This in turn causes the bones and joints to deteriorate. The calcium deficiency can also be connected with other factors, including lack of exercise, excess tea, coffee or chocolate consumption, or exposure to toxic metals like lead. Excessive stress also causes loss of calcium and magnesium.

Other factors which can cause hormonal imbalances include:-

People with liver damage have a problem detoxifying oestrogen.

Some pesticides mimic oestrogen. Molecules which mimic other molecules take up their space and interfere with their functioning.

Meat contains oestrogen which has been used to fatten the animals.

4) Poor lubrication of the joints.

The synovial fluid between the joints keeps them lubricated. To keep the synovial fluid in proper order good nutrition is needed.

5) Bone strain and deformities.

These are often caused by faulty posture. Regular exercise helps to keep the joints supple and strong.

6) Poor diet.

This includes any of these factors:-

A lack of essential vitamins, minerals and essential oils or acids, such as the ones in fish oil or Evening Primrose oil.

An excess of refined sugar.

Too much saturated fat.

Too many stimulants.

Too much protein. This may surprise you, but a high protein diet can lead to calcium deficiency, and this can lead to a calcium/magnesium imbalance. Vegetable protein is of a higher quality than animal protein, so that less is needed to supply the required amount.

7) Disturbed blood sugar control.

There is a link between inflammation and a resistance to insulin. Too much glucose or insulin in the blood is toxic and will trigger inflammatory reactions. A disturbed glucose supply acts as a powerful oxidant. This can cause damage to cells, fatigue, and inflammation. It is possible to restore the balance of insulin; a nutritionist would help with this.

8) An excess of iron in the body.

This can cause pain, swelling and joint destruction. It is important to maintain a balance of all the minerals, not only iron.

9) Electro- and/or Geopathic Stress.

In the book "Safe as Houses?" by David Cowan and Rodney Girdlestone, the authors describe how electro-magnetic fields and earth stresses can contribute to illnesses. When these energies are combined they form "hot spots" to which, if a person is constantly exposed, can cause all kinds of symptoms in the body, including joint pain, rheumatism, headaches, allergies, depression, fatigue, and is even suspected of contributing to cancer.

The electrical causes of stress include the proximity to power and radar stations, T.V. or communications transmitters and electrical sub-stations. The "hot spots" are found where these sub-surface energies are near underground streams.

Other electrical energy which is potentially detrimental to health include domestic appliances. These all emit low-grade radiation and it is best not only to switch them off when not in use but also to pull plugs out of sockets, especially in the bedroom. If there is a flex within three feet of your head this can interfere with brain waves and prevent a good night's sleep.

I myself noticed some time ago that after using the downstairs telephone my joints frequently stiffened up - the longer the conversation the worse I felt! (This still applies). Why one telephone has this effect rather than another I have no idea, except it is nearer the ground, and possible causes of radiation.

Dr. Sidney Macdonald Baker declares that we are all individuals, with a distinctive immunological and biochemical make-up. If the balance of either of these is disturbed, this can interfere with bodily processes and functions, causing physical problems.

Some ways of dealing with inflammation.

These are some of the ways of dealing with inflammation recommended by Dr. Jeffrey Bland, author of "The Twenty Day Rejuvenation Diet".

1) Calm the immune system.
2) Avoid allergens.
3) Take away the source of oxidants.
4) Add antioxidant nutrients. These include vitamins A, C & E, selenium, zinc, magnesium and quercetin.
5) Essential oils e.g.fish oils and evening primrose oil should be waived if there is an excess of oxidants, as

these too can be oxidised and exacerbate the situation. After the balance is restored by adding antioxidants and nutrients, the essential oils should be resumed.

In rheumatoid arthritis the mitochondria (the cells' energy factories) can be damaged. To restore these, nutrients can be taken which would help to rebuild them. There is a long list of these; they are all contained in a supplement called Mitochondrial Resuscitase, available from Nutri (address at end of book), through nutrition practitioners.

The amino acid glutamine helps to heal the gut and rebuild joints. (It also helps to improve the memory!)

Another amino acid, DLPA is a powerful pain-reliever. I have found it absolutely invaluable and have written about it in detail in Chapter 11.

THE IMPORTANCE OF THE MIND

As already described, the subconscious mind has a vast influence on the physical state. It is now commonly accepted that when there are problems here which have not been resolved, this can have adverse and even devastating effects on the body.

Maybe there are long-standing unpleasant memories, or feelings of resentment, anger or fear. In her book, "You Can Heal Your Life," Louise Hay puts forward the idea that arthritis comes from a constant pattern of criticism - of oneself and other people, and that those who do this therefore attract criticism. The reason for this is that they tend to be perfectionists, as Dr. Solomon found in his research. But no-one is ever perfect and we have to settle for being human, with human failings! We have to learn to forgive ourselves and others, to love ourselves and to look at others with the eyes of love.

Any momentary feelings of annoyance, tension, fear, anger, anxiety, judgment, blaming others or any other feelings of a negative type should be faced up to and released - not always an easy task but awareness of the problem can go a long way towards solving it. There is a saying to this effect: To observe how the body is now, look at how the mind was in the past. To see how the body will be in the future, look at how the mind is now.

It is all very well to say "Stop negative thinking," but what do you replace it with? Of course, the answer is that you replace it with a positive thought! I have found from experience that if someone annoys or offends you, if you can send them a thought of love and understanding, then as well as having an effect on the person, it has an effect on yourself! You immediately feel better about that person, and come back into harmony with yourself. With practice, you find that the times you become annoyed or offended become less and less frequent, because compassion becomes a habit, part of your nature. By harbouring feelings of resentment we are only harming ourselves.

Sometimes we need to be willing to change our ways of thinking.

Louise Hay does wonderful work in enabling people to change their thought patterns, to dissolve fears and deal with states of mind which contribute to illness and disease. She declares that every thought we think creates our future, and what we are today is the result of our past thinking. We create our own illnesses. To achieve peace of mind we have to release the past and learn to love and forgive ourselves and others. The things we find most difficult to do are the lessons we most need to learn.

Affirmations to reprogramme the mind are useful. These are new thought patterns which are used to create a state of health, or indeed for any other purpose. They become more potent when repeated using a mirror, looking into your own eyes.

In illness we must be willing to release the *need* to be ill, to let go of the basic reason for our choosing this condition. We could frequently benefit from looking at our belief systems, which are connected with the radical reasons for our illness. Maybe we have developed a pattern of thinking which is hindering us from moving forward.

If we build up enough self-esteem and self-love we can manage our lives without this "prop," the supporter of our disease. So we have to work on ourselves to change our patterns of thinking. With new self-esteem and self-love we are then able to restructure our lives.

In her fascinating book Louise Hay also gives a reference guide showing the connection between mental states and specific physical diseases and conditions. These are not 100% true for everyone, she explains, although they have been found to be 90-95% accurate. They are therefore a useful point of reference to begin the search for the causes of the disease.

Barbara Brennan, in her book "Light Emerging", gives profoundly insightful exercises for self-healing. These are too detailed to describe here but I would strongly recommend the book to anyone suffering from any illness or disease, or to anyone involved with healing in its widest sense.

****

Whatever the causes are, it is possible, with clever management and awareness of the factors which exacerbate the physical symptoms, to enable the suffering of pain and stiffness to be at the absolute minimum, *without* resorting to the use of drugs. I speak from personal experience, as I think the rheumatologists would agree that I was a pretty severe case.

Nevertheless I feel that I have got to the "nitty-gritty" in the management of arthritis, at least for myself, if not for others. However it is an ongoing vigil for I am well aware that if I allow certain factors to lapse, especially with the diet, the pain and stiffness returns, although probably not as severely as it would have done several years ago.

In the natural order of things, we should be in a state of harmony, balance and equilibrium. This does not mean that life should be easy to keep us in this state. On the contrary, we can only develop and grow by meeting and overcoming challenges and problems. But we have to find the peace, harmony and unity within ourselves, and discover how to maintain this state, each of us to remain an integrated human being, able freely to express the deeper self through the mind, feelings and body. It is when we separate ourselves from this unity, this natural equilibrium that we encounter problems.

Once we encounter disease, how do we deal with it?

We have choices. We may choose to "go along" with the drug treatment prescribed by the doctors, following their instructions to the letter and not really thinking about the consequences of long-term drug treatment.

I have already mentioned the reasons why I was so eager to dispense with the drug therapy. A friend of mine who had rheumatoid arthritis for many years actually died indirectly from the side effects of one of the most common drugs prescribed for arthritis, taken over a long period of time. People have no idea what they are risking when they take drug medication. Doctors mainly treat the symptoms and not the cause, and the drugs they prescribe *mask* the pain and stiffness. You therefore tend to be more active than you should be, during a "flare-up", risking further damage to the joints and muscles. For me personally, one of the greatest reasons for dispensing with the drugs is that they pollute the body with rubbish, waste and toxins, in fact producing the opposite effect from what is needed to cleanse the system, a priority for allowing natural healing processes to take place. They therefore hinder, rather than assist healing.

Another choice is available to us. We can begin to take responsibility for our own body, listening to it with a growing awareness of its needs and limitations, and discover the best and most appropriate ways of dealing with our dis-ease. This method of approach is in some ways more difficult, but it is the path to self-knowledge, hopefully bringing a process of gradual improvement, with occasional magical triumphs and leaps forward, and a continuous feeling of being in charge of yourself, your progress and above all, your life.

Sources for this Chapter:-

Detoxification and Healing - Sidney MacDonald Baker, M.D. Published by Keats Publishing Inc., 1997.

Food Intolerance and Food Aversion - A Joint Report of the Royal College of Physicians and the British Nutritional Foundation, April, 1984.

How to Beat Inflammation without Drugs, an I.O.N. Report on Dr. Jeffrey Bland's Masterclass on Inflammation, 1997. Light Emerging, by Barbara Ann Brennan.

Love Your Disease, by Dr.John Harrison.

Maximum Immunity, by Michael A. Weiner, Ph.D.

Optimum Nutrition Magazine, New Year Issue, 1998.

Rejuvenation with Phytonutrition, cassette tape by Dr. Jeffrey Bland, obtainable from I.O.N.

Safe as Houses? by David Cowan and Rodney Girdlestone.

Say No to Arthritis, by Patrick Holford. (I.O.N.)

Uninvited Guests, by Hermann Bueno, M.D.

Why Food Allergy? - A Report by Patrick Holford. (I.O.N.)

CHAPTER 18.
PARASITES AND SOME WAYS
OF DEALING WITH THEM

A parasite is an animal or plant which lives on or within another organism. Many parasites are harmless, but there is a vast number of parasites which are "pathogenic", i.e. harmful to their host. They take food and protection without giving anything back. In fact they actually do damage to the host's body.

Parasitic infections are now so widespread that, according to Anne Louise Gittelman, author of "Guess What Came to Dinner," eight out of ten people are affected with one parasite or another, or even with multiple infections. Millions in the U.K. suffer with digestive complaints caused by parasites, and recent research claims that parasites are responsible for many chronic health problems, including rheumatoid arthritis.

SYMPTOMS OF PARASITICAL INFECTION

There are numerous symptoms, including:-

Irritation of tissues which leads to swelling and inflammation.

Allergic reactions.
Abdominal pains and cramps.
Arthritis.
Autoimmune Diseases.
Chronic Fatigue.
Constipation.
Diarrhoea.
Flatulence.
*Gastritis.
Altered Intestinal Permeability.
Immune System Problems.
Joint and Muscle Aches and Pains.
Sleep Disturbances.

I have included here only the ones which may be relevant in rheumatoid arthritis.There are many more signs of parasitical infection.

*Many years ago I was diagnosed as having gastritis and was prescribed medication which I took for perhaps nine years. I now think that this may have been a parasitical infection which, not properly dealt with, could have been instrumental in precipitating rheumatoid arthritis. There could be a connection here with the following disclosure.

From a recent "stool" test, carried out at Parascope Laboratory, I was found to have the parasite Blastystis Hominis. This ameoba-like organism resides in the lining of the intestinal wall, and is notoriously difficult to eradicate. Its symptoms include irritable bowel, chronic fatigue, and **arthritic and rheumatic complaints.** It has been found in the synovial fluid in the knee of a person with arthritis.

MAJOR SOURCES OF CONTAMINATION.

In Britain there are three main sources:-

1) Through tap water or contaminated food, or surfaces. This would include food which is improperly cooked or stored.
2) Through pets, their faeces and from human faeces, nappies etc.
3) From infection acquired abroad.
4) From surgery and/or tube feeding in hospital.

DIAGNOSIS

Diagnosis may be difficult. N.H.S. hospitals on the whole do not use techniques which can help to identify parasites. People and even many G.P'S are not aware of the extent of parasitical infections. Even though they are so common, there is a lack of detection.

If you wish to discover which parasite(s) you are playing host to, the best plan of campaign would be to contact a qualified practitioner or one of the diagnostic laboratories directly.

The best laboratories for detecting parasites (recommended in the Optimum Nutrition magazine) are:-

Parascope Laboratory. Tel: 0113 292 4657.
Diagnos-Techs Labs. Tel: 0121 458 3407.
Great Smokies Diagnostic Laboratory: through Health Interlink. Tel: 01582 794 094.

The test involves sending samples of stools to be analysed, with several days lapse between samples, for a more complete and thorough diagnosis. On receiving your result, you will probably need assistance from a health care practitioner or qualified nutritionist. I.O.N. can help you to find one locally. (See addresses.)

TREATMENT.

Dr. Jeffrey Bland advises The four "R's":-
Remove
Replace
Re-inoculate
Repair.

The first aim of treatment is to rid the body of all stages of the parasite's life-cycle - adult, egg, ova, cyst etc. The treatment can become more complicated if there is more than one parasite. It can take up to a year to eliminate parasites from the system.

In treating parasite infections, drugs which were once thought to be safe have now been found to have side effects, some of them serious. The best way to deal with them therefore is with herbal preparations.

PARASITES - HERBAL REMEDIES

There is a wide variety of herbal remedies which have anti-parasitical properties. The following list include herbs which can destroy intestinal worms and parasites.

Garlic - prevents and fights infection from yeast, fungus, bacteria, viruses and protozoa; also against tapeworms, roundworms, pinworms and hookworms. Generally non-toxic but can cause irritation to intestines, and also dermatitis.

Black Walnut hull - anti-fungal, antiviral, antiworm and antibacterial. Not for infants or small children.

Chinese Wormwood - protozoa e.g. giardia, yeast, liver fluke and blood fluke. Can be used with:-

Grapefruit Seed Extract (Citricidal) - effective against 800 bacteria and virus strains, 100 strains of fungi as well as a great number of parasites.

Wormwood - pinworms, roundworms, threadworms.

Goldenseal - protozoa and roundworms.

Turmeric - fungus e.g. candida; E.coli.

Clove - anti-microbe, antifungal, antibacteria. Kills parasite eggs. Promotes digestion & eliminates gas.

Sage & Thyme - intestinal worms. Should not be used in large amounts. Fungal infections e.g. athletes foot & skin parasites e.g. scabies, crabs and lice - use externally (tincture or oil).

Fennel seed - helps to remove waste material & parasites from body,. The oil can cause skin irritation, nausea and other side-effects.

Artemisia - effective against worms.

Ginger - against roundworms, blood-fluke & fish roundworm larvae. Also against protozoa Trichomonas Vaginalis. Also for dog heartworm. Useful for digestive upsets.

Tansy leaves - against worms in children . Care should be taken not to overdose, which can cause nausea, diarrhoea, etc.

Gentian root - for digestive disorders. Effective against Entamoeba Hystolica. Expels intestinal worms.

Cayenne - digestive disorders. Kills parasites. Do not use if an ulcer is present, or chronic bowel irritation.

Angelica - especially for protozoa Trichomonas. Do not use in pregnancy.

Pumpkin seeds - paralyses worms but does not kill them, so also take something to move the worms. The seeds are useful for people or children who cannot take stronger herbs. Eating them regularly may help to prevent worms.

Quassia chips - use externally for head lice, fleas and scabies.

If you normally take glutathione, you should abstain from it while taking treatment for parasite infection; this applies especially to artemisia.

Choosing which herbs to use depends on the type of infection, but you can buy preparations which combine several of the above.

To replace and re-inoculate the system, acidopholus and bifidus bacteria are best. These help to balance the intestinal flora and prevent further infection.

To repair the gut, nutrients including vitamin E, zinc, pantothenic acid, and glutamine are recommended.

PREVENTION

To prevent re-infestation of the parasite there are many measures you can take. Here are some steps to prevent parasitical infections.

1) Drink filtered, boiled or bottled water.
2) Eat organic, spray-free food, but wash it thoroughly.
3) Wash hands with soap before meals; use a nailbrush to clean under fingernails.
4) Support the immune system by taking antioxidants.
5) Cook food at the correct temperature:- 180 degrees to kill parasites and bacteria. Meat - at least 325 degrees;

bake fish at 400 degrees, 8-10 minutes per inch of thickness.

6) Beware of raw foods such as sushi. Japan, China and Korea have a high incidence of infection from raw fish.
7) Sanitise all toilet seats and bowls, especially those used by children.
8) Don't walk barefoot, especially in moist, sandy soil.
9) To clean contact lenses, use sterilised lens solutions, not tap water.
10) Keep small children away from puppies and kittens which have not been regularly dewormed, and don't let them kiss animals.

The best line of defence is a strong, healthy immune system.

MEDICINE OF THE FUTURE (?)

In the summer of 1998 I read a book "The Cure for All Diseases", by Dr. Huelda Regher Clark, in which the author described a machine which kills parasites connected with causing diseases.

After six years of intensive research carried out in the U.S.A. Dr.Clark came to the conclusion that *all* diseases are primarily caused by *parasites* and/or *pollutants*. Her exciting research included a discovery that all living things emit electrical impulses which vibrate at specific frequencies. Of course this includes human beings but we vibrate at a much higher rate.

Dr. Clark found that if she ran an extremely low voltage through the bandwidth which included the organisms she was able to eradicate them completely! From this research, a simple hand-held machine was devised, known as a "Frequency Generator" or "Zapper". I decided to purchase one.

To illustrate some of Dr. Clark's findings:-

Dr. Clark had discovered that everyone with certain forms of cancer contained the human intestinal fluke in their livers. Everyone with asthma had Ascaris (cat and dog worms) in their lungs, and everyone with diabetes had pancreatic fluke of cattle.

Arthritis was mentioned and this tied in with what I already knew - that I was housing a parasite called Blastocystis Hominis. So I began using the "Zapper" on a regular basis.

The machine has two copper handles to hold and you "zap" three times, for seven minutes each time, with an interval of at least twenty minutes between each zap. The first zap supposedly kills the parasites. But when they die they release *their* parasites into the body So further zapping is required. There is a warning that the machine is not suitable for anyone with a heart condition and/or pacemaker, or pregnant mothers.

In the space of several months two more machines came into my life. One, a machine which works like acupuncture, (without the use of needles) was introduced to me by a neighbour who had used it for long-standing back problems, with good results. I bought one to use especially for the right knee, which was still troublesome at times.

After each treatment the knee showed an improvement and no longer bothered me at night. (At the same time I had started taking DLPA - please see Chapter 11.)

The other machine, which was much more expensive, came from the U.S.A. This one was a more sophisticated version of the Zapper and I shall describe it in more detail, as I think it is an extremely important device.

The machine is about nine inches square and, like the Zapper there are two cylinder-shaped hand-holds. Unlike the Zapper, which uses batteries, this one can be plugged into the mains supply. On the machine are number buttons. In the extremely informative handbook are shown the numbers of the different frequencies of the organisms connected with each condition or disease. You key in the appropriate numbers and switch on.

The advantage of this Bio-frequency instrument over the Zapper is that it is very specific. The accuracy of each resonant frequency in the instrument is designed to match the frequency of the targeted organism. In the handbook are listed numerous conditions, each with a series of frequency numbers, which are keyed in according to your condition. You sit holding the metal handles while the process runs through the numbers, one minute on each at first; you may progress to two or three minutes later on. There is a frequency monitor which you can control so that you can just feel a slight vibration. The strength of the vibrations may vary, so you have to be aware when the numbers change, to monitor it. Some frequencies are stronger than others! There are also metal plates (contained in fabric "sleeves") which are placed under the feet. This passes the vibrations through the lower part of the body.

For general arthritis there are fourteen numbers so the treatment lasts about a quarter of an hour, on one minute per number. As you progress, the programmes are increased to two then three minutes.

After the treatment you have to drink a considerable amount of water each day for several days, as when the organisms die off, they release *their* toxins into the body. This can cause adverse reactions including headache, increased pain, diarrhoea, etc. The water helps to eliminate the toxins.

Results

On September 24th 1998 at a friend's house I used the Bio-frequency machine for the first time, on the general arthritis programme. On the way home my knees started to throb and I began to feel a headache coming on. So I drank some spring water from the small bottle I always carried around with me. This temporarily alleviated the headache. During the rest of that day I was to feel soreness, aches and pains in the joints and muscles, which seemed to travel from one part of my body to another, even in places where I did not know I had a problem! So I drank water continually. I was not looking forward to the night!

Before I went to sleep I took a detox tablet and was surprised to find I had a good night - the most comfortable I had experienced for a long time. Next day I had very little pain.

I soon realised that a lot depended on what I ate; if I "slipped up" by eating too much of the "wrong" sorts of food, I would suffer the usual discomfort and pains in the familiar places such as the knees, elbows and so on.

Each time I used the machine I had some sort of reaction, usually a headache which was relieved by drinking water. Sometimes the reaction was quite severe; this was also the experience of two arthritic friends who also used the machine. But within two or three days this response was always followed by an improvement in the condition, often quite marked.

I was cautiously excited by my progress. About the same time as I had begun using the machine I had also started taking DLPA and I felt sure that this too was instrumental in my dramatic improvement. However the the danger of feeling so *well* was that I would be tempted to eat some delicious little "treats" such as chocolate raisins, Greek yoghourt, etc. This was not always wise because once again the old familiar pain would return.

I had to realise that I must still be aware of ongoing food problems, in spite of feeling generally so much better.

Another machine came into my life much more recently. This is the InterX machine, as described in Chapter 11. At present all I can say is that it appears to be remarkably successful in dealing with arthritic aches and pains. I have high hopes for its future in the West!

Candida seemed to be my greatest problem, the symptoms including pain at the right side of my head and right ear. The programmes on the machine all ended with the number 28 for candida, and after using it I felt the usual symptoms. One day it was so severe that I drank about four litres of water up to bedtime, to help alleviate it.

Having a problem in the liver I followed the "liver programme" on January 16th. for the first time. This provoked the usual headache and also intermittent pain in the region of the liver, which lasted until the next day, when I felt something *shift* in that area - as though releasing something. This happened twice then the pain vanished. The next day I felt very well with hardly any pain at all.

I have to say that I still use the machine on a regular basis - about once a week. Although the improvement has been maintained, I cannot say if my condition would deteriorate if I stopped using it.

My thanks go to Antony Haynes for his informative article on parasites in the Optimum Nutrition magazine, Volume 11 No.1.

Other sources:-

The Cure for all Diseases, by Dr. Huelda Regher Clark.

Detoxification and Healing, by Sidney MacDonald Baker, M.D.

Maximum Immunity, by Michael A. Weiner, Ph.D.

Uninvited Guests, by Hermann Bueno, M.D.

Cassette tape:- Rejuvenation with Phytonutrition, a Public Lecture by Dr. J. Bland, I.O.N., 1997.

CHAPTER 19.
SELF-HEALING - SUMMARY

This book has been something of a mixture, an amalgamation of experience and discoveries in the realm of self-healing and healing therapies. I sincerely hope that you have not found it too disjointed, naive or simplistic. Several years ago, when I mentioned to Dr.Patel the fact that I was writing a book about my experiences, he advised, "Write it simply, so that ordinary people can understand it."

"Manny", I replied, "It's the only way I can write!"

In order to help alleviate arthritis, I have delved into all kinds of possible means of help and discovered some interesting things on the way. I am not suggesting that you (if you are a "sufferer") do the things I have done. I suppose I have always been a bit of a rebel; the more unusual and less obvious have always held fascination for me, and my curiosity has often led me off the beaten track. When walking in the woods, if I arrive at a fork in the path, with one way beaten down and well-trodden, the other way covered with autumn leaves, I have always tended to choose the leafy one. However, if you choose the path which is less-trodden, it is necessary to be aware of the hidden hazards and pitfalls.

The way I chose to take has constituted a marathon of trial with occasional "error". (If you believe in error!) Some of the therapies have been incredibly successful, others perhaps less so, but *all* have contributed something in the way of knowledge and experience.

Self-healing is hard work. For me it has been a long process, which is still continuing. There have been setbacks and sometimes I have wondered if it is worth all the effort, but now, I can categorically say that, for myself, it has been worth every

bit of the time, money and energy expended on it. In spite of some not inconsiderable hiccoughs along the way, the rewards when another step has been achieved has made the whole thing worthwhile.

The good news is that there seem to be basic guidelines in the management and improvement of rheumatoid arthritis which *anyone* can follow. I am not going to suggest that you choose this way, but here are the methods which I have used in order to return to health.

The first thing to do is to take personal responsibility for your body. No-one knows your body better than you; its needs are essential to your comfort and well-being. The opposite to dis-ease is *ease*. This does not mean you should sit at home watching T.V. and eating chocolates all afternoon! No, the sort of needs I am talking about are ones like the right foods to eat, regular exercise, fresh air and sufficient rest. Responsibility for yourself implies that you learn what is *best* for your body. It is a matter of balance in all things.

The second matter to address is to look at anything which may be hindering your progress back to harmony.

Sometimes it would be beneficial to change our environmental circumstances, -the way we live (or even who we are living with!). This may involve enormous changes in our lives and is not always easy or practical. If we cannot change our situation, as Saint Francis said, we have to accept it, with grace.

More often, perhaps, we need to address our state of mind and look at the *real* causes of our attitudes and thinking. Any negativity, such as fear, resentment, anger or anxiety should be dealt with, as stated in previous chapters.

If we are holding onto anger and resentment we may have to be willing to *forgive*. We should think back to events in our lives to see *who* we have to forgive. As well as forgiving others, we need to forgive *ourselves*.

It is absolutely necessary for us to release the past in order for the healing process to begin and develop.

If the feelings date from childhood we may have to be willing to forgive our parents. Even if they are long deceased it is necessary to come to terms with a feeling of forgiveness in the heart, in order to free oneself from the bonds of deep-down anger and resentment. This releasing is an incredibly therapeutic thing to do and can often be the precursor to a change of outlook, bringing a wonderful feeling of grace, which actually facilitates the healing process. *Affirmations* are a great help with this. Louise Hay suggests:-

"I forgive you for not being the way I wanted you to be. I forgive you and I set you free."

The next thing in a disease such as arthritis, is to be as pure and clean of toxins and poisons as it is possible to be, maybe by regular detoxification or other methods described in the book. Also it is important to discover if you have a parasite or parasites which may have a bearing on your condition, even being the main cause. If you find this to be the case, the problem needs addressing by means described in Chapter 18.

There is no specific way for people to detoxify themselves; it depends on the individual. Arnold Ehret did it by fasting. Dr. Norman Walker advises colonic irrigations; the Arthritic Association method entails taking detoxification tablets, with fasting, one day a week. The Gerson Therapy advocates enemas, fasting and juice therapy. This last way, the Gerson Therapy, was the one I chose for the initial cleansing, but on a regular basis I now follow the Arthritic Association programme of weekly Detox tablets followed by a fruit and vegetable juice fast the following day. This appears to be sufficient to rid the body of toxic waste material on a regular basis.

Once cleansed, the person needs to be vigilant about what they eat, drink and inhale into their bodies. The diet in arthritis is of paramount importance. It is necessary to find the foods which suit you and avoid the ones which cause you pain and stiffness. Allergies may be a key factor in your condition. As described in the book, it is possible to discover what is affecting you, by various means of testing. Candida too is more common than people realise. Dramatic improvements can often be made by changing diet.

It is important that food should be top-grade, natural food, as fresh as possible. Think of your body as a machine - perhaps your car. It needs fuel and water. You wouldn't put inferior grade fuel and contaminated water into your car, would you? But some people treat their bodies with this sort of lack of care. They look after their cars better than they look after their bodies! It doesn't seem very sensible. Your body will hopefully be with you long after your car has become obsolescent. You can get a new car but you can't get a new body! Not in this lifetime, anyway, in spite of the latest advances in technology!

So the food you put into your precious, irreplaceable body should be uncontaminated by additives, pesticides, colourings or other chemicals, as far as it is possible to ascertain. The diet should be mainly alkaline, preferably following food combining principles of not mixing starch and protein in the same meal, and consisting mostly of fresh salads, fruit and vegetables, especially dark green leaves, preferably raw, and organic if possible. Vegetable juice is helpful, made on a juice machine. This way of eating becomes a habit, bringing awareness of the purpose of food, and enjoyment of the taste of the pure, natural goodness of it.

In connection with food and digestion, it is advisable to be aware of a very much overlooked part of your body, your colon! As already described, many people are not aware that they are walking around carrying pounds and pounds of caked-on, toxic material inside their colons. This is why the cleansing is so necessary.   Constipation can herald disease and prevent progress as already stated. On a daily basis it should be avoided at all costs by keeping the bowels "regular." The fruit and vegetables will help with this. If you know or suspect you are constipated, you can deal with it by following the advice given below. Having said that, it is best not to depend on external ways to treat it; natural ways of correct eating should keep your colon in good order and bowel habits regular.

If, once cleansed, a problem arises with pain and stiffness which inhibits movement and causes discomfort, in my experience this is usually due to either a problem in the intestinal tract, such as constipation; or because of incompatible eating - eating "foods which fight"; or ingesting some chemical or other. Another reason is overstrain of muscles and joints, so it is important to be constantly aware of one's limitations. Yet another reason is tiredness, so sufficient rest is required. As has been emphasised in several places throughout this book, listening to the body teaches us what we need to do.

To alleviate an attack of pain, stiffness or constipation without resorting to drugs I do one of the following:-

1. Take Detox tablets. These work overnight and you feel better the next morning. This method is really part of the weekly fasting process recommended by the Arthritic Association, but sometimes I take them when I know the pain is connected with something I have eaten.

2. Take an enema of warm boiled water (Blood temperature). This clears the bowel and colon and usually brings instant relief.

3. Take Dr. Mansfield's remedy. (See Chapter 6, Testing for Allergies.) This has an effect within a short time, maybe in as little as half-an-hour. Another dose may be taken six hours later.

4. In cases which are not too severe, and which are definitely connected with food, especially a recent meal, Swedish Bitters is a useful remedy. Another one, Aloe Vera, may be taken at bedtime, although first thing in the morning is preferable as it should normally be taken on an empty stomach.

Food supplements including herbal remedies have played an enormous part in my progress. The tablets supplied by the Arthritic Association, especially the detoxifying ones have been invaluable, as well as other ones, such as "K Compound" for the potassium.

Specific herbal remedies recommended by the kinesiologist have helped with candida, dysbiosis (imbalance of the intestinal flora), and the liver problem, among other things, and I am indebted to Ralph Pike for his skill.

To boost the immune system, two excellent herbal remedies are Echinacea and Quercetin, as described in Chapter 11.

Vitamins and minerals play an essential part in a healing programme for arthritis. (Also in Chapter 11). Many people are deficient in all sorts of nutrients and need supplementation, but even on an ongoing basis they are invaluable to provide the necessary requirements for our bodies, especially for people suffering from conditions such as arthritis. I have personally found that my energy level has increased since I started to take vitamin and mineral supplements. The juice too adds to your energy level.

As already stated, both Aloe Vera and Swedish Bitters have helped tremendously. I cannot *prove* this. I just know that, since I started taking them regularly, or rather when needed in the case of Swedish Bitters, I have felt better in a general way. One of the effects of both these products, because of their capacity to facilitate the digestive processes, is to make you feel *really* comfortable inside. Their other properties too are extremely beneficial and you find you are able to eat a wider range of foodstuffs without ill-effects.

Complementary therapies are auxiliary aids in one's progress, but they can only work for you if you are prepared to aid the process by also working on yourself, by diet and the other things I have mentioned. Some of these practices, such as massage and shiatsu, become a way of life to be used regularly; they can be utilised daily if necessary, or you may wish to visit a qualified practitioner for a thorough session, if you can afford it. Other therapies, such as reflexology, acupuncture, massage, Alexander Technique and chiropractic are of great benefit as and when they are required. There are numerous methods of help available nowadays which offer all kinds of treatment according to your need (and pocket!).

Other necessary factors in self healing are regular exercise, correct breathing and fresh air. I cannot over- emphasise the importance of breathing properly. It enables the body to perform as it should and facilitates a relaxed frame of mind which in turn has a beneficial physiological effect on the body. Different types of breathing may be used for different purposes; one type is used in relaxation, another for re-energising yourself. It is really exciting when you discover the power of breathing!

Walking is excellent as it combines exercise, breath and fresh air. If you can, set aside some time each day to walk, preferably under trees so that you inhale plenty of oxygen, and you will soon feel the benefit in increased energy, stamina and mobility.

Other regular exercise might include swimming, if you can do it. This is said to be the best complete exercise you can do, as it involves the whole of your body. Chi Kung or Tai Chi are excellent; they are simple to do but hold countless benefits to the body, mind and spirit. Dancing is wonderful too, especially free, undirected dancing. Also recommended are Circle Dancing, Five-Rhythm Dancing and Dances of Universal Peace. Even if you have only ten minutes to spare, you could put on a tape and dance around the room, or do some Chi Kung. This makes an enormous difference to how you feel, on all levels.

Two additional powerful self-healing therapies are singing, and laughing! Having fun is very important. It is not necessary to join a singing group, -just singing around the house while doing chores is therapeutic.

All these things, dancing, singing and laughter have a beneficial effect on the immune system and are so important for our well-being. I personally find that listening to music helps to keep me in a harmonious state of mind.

Really I want to say that all these things are ideally a manifestation of something else. That is, they are an expression of a *deeper* you, the real you. They are wonderful ways of expressing how you are, deep down inside; being "in touch" with yourself. They then become a way of life which symbolises your most profound feelings. Expressing our essence, our deepest selves is probably the most healing thing we can do.

Sometimes temporary emotional problems can cause setbacks, which interrupt your progress towards wholeness and harmony. Stress or tension connected with these problems can be dealt with by expressing yourself in such activities as the singing and dancing, also in shouting and crying, or even sex! Any of these things can bring relief; it is a matter of personal inclination (and perhaps opportunity!). It is vitally imperative to express any feelings; the harmful effects when you suppress them have been described earlier in this chapter. Once again I wish to emphasise that the suppression of emotional feelings prevents you from being deeply relaxed inside, which is a prerequisite to healing. I read recently of a study among some women who were given the opportunity to express their feelings once a fortnight. Despair, rage and fear were freely allowed to be expressed. This group of women lived twice as long as those who did not have such an opportunity.

You may however have a problem which is continuous and which you cannot see any method of solving in the foreseeable future. If this is the case, one way of dealing with it, or at least making it easier to cope with, is to live *absolutely in the present moment,* as outlined in Chapter 16. This way of looking at things takes some practice, but is well worth doing. It means you do not think about the past or the future...you stop mulling over past traumas and events and you also cease to feel anxious about the future.

To do this practice you just concentrate completely on whatever you are doing *right now,* in this instant. This may be difficult at first, but with practice it becomes easier to achieve. Of course, you have to make necessary plans and arrangements, but apart from that, just be aware of the *here and now.* Living in the present means that we take every event as it comes and accept every person without judging or criticising.

A spin-off from this practice is that it concentrates the mind wonderfully, giving clarity and increased enjoyment to your activities, as there are no clouds to obscure your vision. The most simple and ordinary things suddenly become incredibly meaningful.

Other help in dealing with ongoing problems comes in the form of yoga, relaxation and meditation.

I have already described the part that both yoga and meditation have played in my progress; the healing meditations described in Chapter 9 have been of immeasurable importance in my progress and I still practise them nearly every day. The power of them has to be experienced to be believed! In both meditation and relaxation the immune system is activated, enabling you to reach a point where you feel so euphoric...you could purr like a cat! Affirmations, too, are extremely potent in training the mind to see everything in a positive light, reprogramming ones attitudes, and so helping in the natural healing processes. It has now been scientifically proved that positive thinking actually stimulates production of substances called cytokines in the brain, which boost the immune system. This in turn aids recovery from disease.

The meaning of "to suffer" is "to allow". So if we are allowing disease to be present in our body, by the same token we can say, "No, I won't allow it!" You can refuse to play host or hostess to it. This may be a catalyst to a change in attitude and/or perception.

When you negate something by saying "No", you have to replace it with positive energy. To facilitate this process, one thing you can try is to obtain a picture of the part(s) of your body which are troublesome (manifesting symptoms), whether it is an internal organ, bone, muscle or whatever. The picture should be a clear drawing of a perfectly healthy section of the body.

Sit with the picture for a few minutes and study it until it becomes ingrained in your mind. Then close your eyes and concentrate on that part of your body. Imagine it to be filled with light - complete, whole and perfect. Try to do this for a few minutes each day. This will assist the healing process, which will enable your body to return to a state of harmony and health.

Spiritual healing is frequently very successful. An instantaneous cure is quite rare, but regular contact or absent healing has a beneficial effect. There are healing groups in many towns and cities, where contact healing is given. These include groups run by the National Federation of Spiritual Healers and also White Eagle Lodge, as well as other reputable healing groups. To find your nearest group, please see the addresses and telephone numbers at the end of the book.

Ivan Cooke says:-

"No true healing of soul or body can take place without some corresponding spiritual effort on the part of the patient, but the patient can be helped, his own efforts supplemented; his spirit can be nurtured and strengthened."

You can of course learn to access the healing energies for yourself, (as described in Chapter 9,) and experience the magic of this.

When accessing the "light," we have to remember that we are merely channels for the Divine power to flow through us. Being channels, we can also send the light, the Divine energy, to other people - to friends, family, to people in the world who are suffering in any way, to animals and even to the planet itself, which is suffering at the hands of Mankind. Although we cannot see the energy which is used in this kind of healing, nevertheless it is all around us, and has now been proved to exist. Think of a portable radio, with no wires. You turn the knob, and hear the sound of music. How does that happen? The air is full of all kinds of invisible waves and particles of energy.

This brings me to something which is absolutely crucial to the self-healing process, or indeed, *any* healing process.

Throughout the book I have frequently mentioned the power of the mind. If I had to choose one thing above all others which has made the greatest contribution to my overall improvement I would have to say it is THOUGHT. It is vitally important, when having a potentially long-term health problem, to turn our thoughts away from ourselves, *outwards* towards other people, interests and activities. People who are "wrapped up" in themselves find they will be left alone; their friends will drift away one by one, for who wants to be near a person who is immersed in self-pity, moaning about their complaints? A lively interest in other people and one's surroundings, as well as a sense of humour is vital to our well-being. If you do not have an outside interest, or a purpose in your life, something which is important to you and fills you with enthusiasm or at least a feeling of warmth and happiness, then I suggest it is crucial to your welfare to find one!

Through our *thoughts* we can change our *lives,* bringing ourselves into peace and harmony which lead to the healing of mind, spirit and body. I cannot over-emphasise this.

YOUR THOUGHTS CAN CHANGE YOUR LIFE!

INWARD THINKING	OUTWARD THINKING
Introversion	Hope
Aimlessness	Interest
Self-preoccupation	Friends
Resentment	Involvement
Withdrawal	Purpose
Loneliness	Expansion
Dis-ease	Self-confidence
Depression	Positivity
Stagnation	Fulfilment

Apart from the above, there is a third type of thinking. (There may be more for all I know!) Indeed, it is not so much to do with *thought,* but more a state of *being.* It is to be God-centred, and this is the best of all.

Of course, it depends on what your perception of "God" is - some people's idea of the Divine may be the Universe, the Light or something else. But whatever it is, if you are centred in your conception of God, living in God-consciousness every moment of your life, or at least working towards this highly-evolved state, you do not fall into either of the above categories. Your diagram would be more like this:-

Forgiveness

Dedication

Surrender to a Higher Power.

Universal and Uncondition Love and Compassion

Lightness

Peace

Joy

There is no barrier on this diagram, because you feel "at one" with all that is.

CHANGE BRINGS GROWTH!

To summarise the whole self-healing principles, I cannot better Ivan Cooke's beautiful words:-

"Anything consistently inharmonious in the life may predispose the body to illness... Practise the laws of purity and godliness; eat clean food always; breathe fresh air, drink only pure water and fruit juices; breathe in the great harmonies of nature; rest, sleep and work harmoniously without tension, rush, fear or anxiety; attain and hold fast to that serene and tranquil life lived by all those who have mastered their lower self; don't let your emotional self be consumed by desire and demands; all these must be controlled if you would grow healthy, whole and wise."

And who would not choose to grow healthy, whole and wise?

EPILOGUE

"Your pain is the breaking of the shell that encloses your understanding. Even as the stone of the fruit must break, that its heart may stand in the sun, so must you know pain."

- From "The Prophet", by Khalil Gibran.

In the prologue I described my physical state before I assumed personal responsibility for my body and undertook the healing of it. That time, more than nineteen years ago, is difficult for me to imagine now; I seem to have travelled a million light years since then. But yes, if I think hard, I *do* remember what it was like to have pain as a constant companion; to never feel really comfortable in myself, internally or externally and to suffer from all sorts of minor disorders. Nowadays I have very little pain most of the time, except when I have eaten something which affects me, sometimes inadvertently. Then I have to think hard what I have eaten.

My progress, although sometimes erratic, has on the whole been steady. The mobility has improved beyond all my wildest hopes and dreams; it is so gratifying to walk in comfort, dance and generally move easily and freely.

I have much more energy than previously and generally feel fitter. I am able to work for hours at the computer, or at some artwork, without any increase in discomfort. It is wonderful!

The whole therapy has been for me a tremendous learning process, not only in the management of arthritis, but in the realms of other wonderful and amazing things, in particular the sphere of the mind; also of the spiritual side of myself, which maybe I would not have encountered to such an extent had I not "suffered" with arthritis. Because of these experiences I have to say that I am actually grateful for having had the disease, for it has opened my eyes to different worlds and ways of being, in a most wonderful way. There is an appropriate quotation to describe this:-

"There is no such thing as a problem without a gift to you in its hands. You seek problems because you need their gifts."

- From "Illusions," by Richard Bach.

What wonderful gifts I have received!

Even pain is, or can be a gift, though we may not realise it at the time of suffering. I am not saying that it is a pleasant or agreeable thing to suffer pain, but that it can bring an awareness of all kinds of realisations.

"And could you keep your heart in wonder at the daily miracles of your life, your pain would not seem less wondrous than your joy..."

- Khalil Gibran.

Pain and problems are difficult to cope with unless you have some sort of faith. The more difficulties you have, the more need you have to trust in God, the Universe or whatever is your concept of the Divine.

I am convinced that everyone is cared for and protected by unseen helpers. They are always with you, hoping to be called upon when needed! They provide help in all kinds of ways, with your state of mind as well as in practical purposes. Their tender, loving care has often filled me with humility. Without their help I would have found it immeasurably difficult to cope at times of severe pain, when problems seemed overwhelming. At these times it has been such a relief just to surrender everything, to surrender it all to a Higher Power. When you do this, immediately a burden seems to be lifted from your shoulders.

When I was looking for a quotation to support the above statement, on opening "The Quiet Mind" for inspiration my eye immediately fell on the following passage:-

"Never doubt the power, the wisdom and the love of God."

When you are on "the right track", you don't have to search for what you need; it usually comes to hand!

One of the realities I have learned over the past ten years is that it is not the *problem* that is important but our *attitude* to it. If we look at each "problem" as a challenge, a personal test of our character, if you like, which contains a precious lesson for us to learn, it changes our whole conception of the situation. As stated earlier, the *real* achievements are not what we have *done* during the day, but the way we have dealt with our tasks and difficulties. So the inner growth takes place.

Being aware of the "how" of doing things, rather than what we actually do has brought me the realisation of the importance of *order* in my life. Doing things in an orderly way is a vital and difficult lesson which I am still learning!

It is an important one, nevertheless; from experience I have found that if I "skip" a process, or try to "get away" with not doing things properly, in order to save time, then things go wrong; I have to pay for it later! If I don't put my shoes away, then I fall over them. Or if I try to carry too many bags of shopping from the car into the house, then I drop one (or more!). So now I try to take the time to do things carefully and properly, completing one task before beginning another.

I hope you have found something in the book which is helpful to you, or at least of some interest. I wrote the book because I could not help it. After several years of recording my efforts and progress in large notebooks it seemed the logical thing to do; an inner "voice" encouraged me in this. But over the last few years many people who have noted my improvement with interest have approached me seeking help with their arthritic aches and pains, so this book is really for them, and all the people like them. If even one person has been helped I shall be delighted.

In spite of giving me some headaches, - figuratively speaking, writing the book has given me great enjoyment. Indeed, I enjoy *everything* so much more now; I have such a sense of... if I had to crystallize it into words, I would have to say that I have an increased sense of appreciation; sights, sounds and activities appear magical to me...walking in the woods; a candle glowing in the twilight; the pure sound of music; sunshine on a frosty day; the eddying and swirling of the stream in the park; even just cleaning up my kitchen!

A Chinese sage said,

"I know the joy of a fish in the river, through my own joy walking along the river."

- Chuang Tzu.

Perhaps the most magical thing of all is to become the co-creator of your own life. When this happens, it brings a wonderful sense of freedom and liberation. You feel guided, yes, but you have the choice of following that "inner voice" of wisdom and compassion, which allows you to flow with everything; or to continue in your old patterns of thought, not changing anything or learning very much. If you choose the way of freedom you will find that it brings an amazing feeling of harmony, balance and unity to your life. And inner harmony can bring peace to the Earth! I should like to repeat that:-

INNER HARMONY CAN BRING
PEACE TO THE EARTH!

For when you find the harmony and peace within yourself, then you become in harmony with your friends, family and everyone with whom you come into contact. The ripples of peace and harmony radiate outwards, as when you throw a pebble into a still lake.

If *everyone* were in this state of peace and equilibrium there would be no reason for war. Each person would care for everyone else with love, compassion and understanding, and peace would reign on Earth!

I should like to finish with a passage of prose which has special meaning for me, one which touches me deeply. This beautiful quotation comes from "Om Sankalpa," by Swami Satyananda and I am indebted to my friend Anna for acquainting me with it.

"Shall I fall upon bended knees and wait for someone to bless me with happiness and a life of golden dreams? No, I shall run into the desert of life with my arms open, sometimes falling, sometimes stumbling, but always picking myself up, - a thousand times if necessary....There shall never be a storm that can wash the path from my feet, the direction from my heart, the light from my eyes or the purpose from my life."

APPENDIX 1
USEFUL TIPS

Dealing with pain.

Place a hot or cold pack on painful areas. You can purchase a gel-filled pouch which can be heated or placed in the fridge, or there are the ever-useful frozen peas, which can be wrapped in a tea-towel.

If parts of the body feel painful and sore, take a hot shower and direct the water onto the painful areas. After some minutes turn the control to "cold" and direct the water onto the same places. Finish off with a cool shower all over, as cold as you can stand it (if you don't have a heart condition), especially on your face. This is wonderful for the circulation, toning up the body, making you feel immensely buoyant and giving you a glow!

If you have pain in legs, ankles, knees or feet, the hot and cold foot plunges as advised by the Arthritic Association are extremely effective in reaching the parts that other therapies cannot reach! (Please see Appendix 3.) If done at bedtime, it seems to induce a good night's sleep.

If knees are painful, try swinging! Going on a swing in a local park is excellent for the knees; it is best to do it during schooltime!

If hands and arms are painful, at bedtime run water into the wash-basin, as hot as you can stand it, then submerge hands and arms as deeply as you are able.

Also at bedtime, taking celery juice helps to alleviate arthritic aches and pains. Put two or three sticks of celery through the juice machine and top with boiling water.

If you like to wear trousers and have problems with painful knees, you often find that the inflammation is made worse because your knees are too warm. Here is a way of keeping your knees cooler than the rest of your legs, especially in cold weather. Cut a pair of thick tights across, at the place where the knees would be. You then have "breeks" and also a pair of long socks. These are nice and warm to wear under your trousers but the knees remain cooler.

Walking on grass rather than on hard surfaces reduces jarring of the knees and hips.

The inspirational Ram Dass, who became disabled after suffering a stroke, was unable to turn in bed by himself. He found that the best way to deal with discomfort and pain is to relax into it, saying "I accept you, pain." This may be difficult at first, but becomes easier with practice.

Shopping.

When shopping, or otherwise, try to carry only one heavy thing at a time, e.g. from the car, even if it means more journeys to and fro.

Also when shopping, using a bag with a strap which goes right round the body saves carrying and avoids strain on the arms. If you *do* have to carry something, use both arms rather than one and support it from underneath.

In department stores, using the lift or escalator will save strain on weight bearing joints.

At home.

All sorts of aids and gadgets are available from the Occupational Therapy Department of your local hospital. Some items, e.g. hand-rails for stairs, or raised toilet seats are usually available at Social Services Departments.

Sit if possible to prepare vegetables, etc.

With arthritic hands, wear wrist splints to prepare vegetables or perform any task which causes pain or strain to the hands or wrists. Wearing the splints in bed at night will help to prevent further deformity.

To save strain on joints when preparing food, buy a food-processor, if you can afford it. Before purchasing, check how easy the controls are to use.

To open tins, use a wall can-opener, or electric tin-opener.

To open jars, there are gadgets available. One which generally "does the trick" successfully is a metal V-shape with jagged sides. Use a damp cloth to hold the jar while you open it.

Levers on taps are useful.

Use two hands to hold cups. At home I always use a light plastic cup.

Pick-up sticks are indispensable if you drop items on the floor, also for reaching things from the back of the fridge, etc. I have two, one for upstairs and one for downstairs.

If you have difficulty walking, an indoor trolley is extremely useful. It helps to steady you and therefore avoid falling. You can keep a pick-up stick on the handle in case of dropping things!

To help with putting on underwear and trousers, a stick with a hook in the end is extremely useful.

Back fastening bras can be fastened at the front and then turned round, or sewn up at the back and a new front-fastening made. There are a number of aids available for dressing. A useful book which describes these is "The Arthritis Helpbook" (Please see Bibliography).

General Hints

Lie flat every day for at least twenty minutes. Lying on the stomach is excellent, especially if you have had hip replacements.

Avoid keeping in one position for a long time. Our natural state is *movement*.   But regular rest is important, too. Try to balance activity and rest.

Always be aware of your position and posture. Think about the position you are resting in -try to keep the body balanced and avoid tension in any part.

APPENDIX 2
CANDIDA

Candida Albicans is a yeast type of organism, yeasts being part of the family of moulds. The systemic infection of the body by this organism is known as candidiasis, or, as it is commonly referred to, candida.

Yeasts normally live on the skin, in the digestive tract and in the ascending colon. In our bodies there is a delicate balance between the yeasts and the bacteria. These micro-organisms produce their own antibiotics and therefore control each other to produce the balance, which keeps us healthy. It is when this equilibrium is disturbed that an overgrowth of a particular organism such as Candida Albicans may occur. This is what happens to cause candidiasis.

Candidiasis causes a wide range of symptoms and conditions, including the following:- Depression; irritability; heartburn; bloating; allergies; migraine; thrush; P.M.T.; anxiety; indigestion; fatigue; acne; cystitis; herpes; sugar and other carbohydrate cravings; alcohol cravings; joint pains; muscle pains; M.E.; Multiple Sclerosis. There are many more.

The Causes of Candidiasis

Antibiotics, which are commonly and frequently prescribed for infections. They kill bacteria including the protective ones that live in the gut and on the skin. This disturbs the balance of the microflora and allows different organisms to overgrow, such as Candida Albicans.

The outcome of this over-use has been an increase in the number of women with thrush. Fortunately it is now recognised that antibiotics have often been used indiscriminately and over-liberally, so the usage is beginning to decrease.

Antibiotics have also been added to animal feed to promote the growth in some farm animals such as pigs, cows and chickens. This also has had an effect on the health of consumers, but now that people have become aware of the problem this practice, in Europe at least, has diminished considerably.

Steroidal treatment also creates imbalances in the intestinal flora, as also does hormone therapy.

Diabetics are prone to candidiasis, due to high blood sugar levels.

A problem is caused when taking **immune-suppressing drugs**. A large proportion of AIDS patients die from candidiasis.

Multiple pregnancies has also been connected with an overgrowth of candida albicans.

Toxins. One indirect cause of candidiasis is the production of a toxin called acetyldehyde. This is produced in the liver, through the fermentation of sugar by yeast, which then forms alcohol. A severe proliferation of candida can produce enough alcohol to make you feel "spaced out" and have difficulty focussing, in fact manifesting the classic symptoms of drunkenness and a hangover.

What causes the symptoms?

Candida produces toxic waste material and this causes a strain on the kidneys and liver, whose function it is to eliminate waste. Larger amounts of nutrition are needed to cope with the metabolism of these toxins, which, if not properly eliminated, circulate round the system, causing the symptoms.

The toxic by-products from candida can damage the intestinal wall. Moreover, because of the conflict between candida and the beneficial bacteria in the gut, pathogenic bacteria are allowed to proliferate as well.

One especially destructive class of bacteria is called the polyamines, which are produced by the incomplete breaking down of undigested proteins. The effects of polyamines have been linked with arthritis and also with the skin disease psoriasis.

The stress on the liver caused by overwork, trying to detoxify the body of uncountable toxins from candida and harmful bacteria, can cause sensitivities to chemicals. Normally a healthy liver can process these easily, but a depleted one is not able to function adequately.

When conditions are ripe for candida proliferation it changes from a yeast to a fungal form, with long root-like mycelia (tendrils). These mycelia can penetrate the mucous membrane lining of the intestinal wall, creating a condition of over-permeable mucosa, commonly called "leaky gut". This condition is thought to be responsible for many disorders, including food intolerances.

Irritation of the mucosa, (intestinal lining) can also lead to "leaky gut". One reason for this is the reaction of the immune system to yeast cells and any parasites which implant themselves in the intestinal wall.

In "leaky gut" condition, instead of all the food being digested in the normal way, proteins can enter the circulation through the minute sieve-like holes. This provokes the immune system again to react to the foreign bodies, which explains why candida sufferers tend to have multiple food intolerances. These often disappear as the candida problem is overcome.

Another manifestation of candidiasis is that spores are released into the circulation by way of the hyphae (tendrils) and the candida can then infiltrate other body parts, including the liver, adrenal glands, lungs and even the nervous system.

There is a condition known as "die-off," which can occur as a result of treatment. Normally the candida cells release their metabolites in a controlled manner. When they are suddenly "hit" with an aggressive therapy they will begin to die. When this happens the cells burst open, releasing their entire contents in one go. This causes a sudden rise in the level of toxins in the body, and therefore a corresponding rise in symptoms.

Doctors normally prescribe drugs such as Nystatin, which is believed to be effective against candida. However, this drug cannot be absorbed into the system, so although it will certainly kill some of the candida within the intestinal tract, it cannot deal with other candida infections. This means that on ceasing treatment the problem will return in full force as the intestinal tract is repopulated from outside.

Another drug, Ketoconazole, is absorbed from the digestive tract and is carried in the bloodstream to the rest of the body, so it will treat candida in the vagina, skin or any other tissues. There is a drawback to this drug though as its safety over a long period of use has not been demonstrated. In fact it can cause damage to the liver, and regular blood tests have to be performed if it is taken for more than a few weeks.

What does the non-orthodox treatment consist of?

The cornerstone of candida therapy is the diet. To grow yeast cultures you need sugar. It is the same with candida. If you deprive it of the sugar it needs to survive it will die.

Sugar is a simple carbohydrate, which is easily absorbed by the candida organisms. Other forms of sugar which come in this category include:-

glucose
fructose (fruit sugar)
dextrose
fruits and fruit juices
lactose (milk sugar)
molasses
maple syrup
corn syrup

It is advisable to read the labels on food packets and tins before purchasing. There are many hidden pitfalls and some people are not aware that dextrose, for instance, is a form of sugar.

Some people may be concerned at omitting energy-producing sweet foodstuffs, and of course, we need some carbohydrates in our diet. Complex carbohydrates are less attractive to the yeast, so these are the ones which we should eat. The more common and accessible ones include:-

cereals; grains (such as wheat, rice, oats, rye, barley, corn, millet)

beans/legumes

potatoes

nuts and seeds.

Re-inoculating the bowel with acid-producing bacteria discourages the growth of the yeast in the intestines. Supplements containing these are referred to as **probiotics**. The most important ones for candidiasis are:-

Lactobacillus acidophilus and lactobacillus bulgaris, and Bifidobacterium bifidum.

These are available in powder or capsules.

Other supplements and foodstuffs which help to eradicate the overgrowth include:-

Echinacea, described in Chapter 11.

Milk thistle (Silymarin). This possesses remarkable liver-protective properties, and provides additional protection against candida overgrowth in the small intestine.

Digestive Enzymes. These are useful in that they help to reinstate proper digestion and control candida overgrowth.

Antioxidants, especially vitamins A, C and E, selenium, zinc and beta carotene. These are vital for the proper functioning of the immune system.

B Vitamins. A deficiency of B vitamins is common in candidiasis. Biotin is a B vitamin. The yeast form of candida changes to the fungal form partly because of a biotin deficiency. So when biotin is added to the diet it can prevent the conversion of the yeast to the fungal form. Biotin is found in pig's kidney, pig's liver and, for vegetarians, wheat bran. **Oleic acid**, contained in olive oil and linseed oil, also seems to prevent this conversion.

Caprylic acid. An anti fungal substance which can be used to great effect. It is extremely safe and is retailed as a food supplement. The effects of it can be enhanced by taking Lactobacillus acidophilus at the same time. This however is only effective within the intestinal tract and is not a systemic treatment, so re-infection can occur.

Garlic.   A highly effective anti-fungal herb. This has to be the whole garlic, not the odourless variety, as the anti-fungal agent contained in it is the allicin which also causes the odour.

Live yoghourt. This contains the beneficial lactobacillus bacteria, which help to prevent an overgrowth of candida albicans in the system. For people who are intolerant to cow's milk, soya yoghourt with live cultures are available.

Some harmful foodstuffs include:-

Anything containing sugar. This includes biscuits, cakes, etc. Many tinned foods include sugar, e.g. baked beans. Always read the small print.

Alcohol. Anything which is fermented, including alcohol, is definitely not advisable for people with candidiasis. Moreover, beer, wine and spirits constitute concentrated carbohydrates, which candida love to consume. Even a small amount of alcohol will produce adverse symptoms in a person with candidiasis.

Vinegar is a fermented food so it is best avoided. Other foods in this category include ketchup, salad dressings, sauerkraut, soya sauce and miso.

Yeast. Any form of yeast can provoke a sensitivity reaction and cause food intolerances which will further weaken the immune system. All forms of yeast should be avoided. Also in this category are mushrooms, mouldy cheese and any foods which have a "bloom" on them, maybe left over foods which have been kept in the refrigerator.

Dairy produce. Lactose in milk feeds candida. Both lactose and casein, a protein also found in milk, are responsible for milk intolerance. Cheeses tend to be susceptible to mould; in any case cheese is a "high risk" food for people with arhritis.

Supplements which help to heal "Leaky Gut" include:-

Goldenseal. This contains a substance called berberine, which blocks certain enzymes which contribute to increased gut permeability. These enzymes include histamine and tyramine.

Citrus seed extract.

Quercetin - a natural bioflavenoid. Quercetin is described in Chapter 11.

Glutamine. This both helps to prevent and reverse a damaged intestinal mucosa.

Ginkgo biloba. Helps to prevent damage and protects intestinal mucosa.

Antioxidants
Vitamin A
Essential fatty acids
Zinc; magnesium
Vitamin B6
Biotin.

A combination of herbal treatment may be used to treat leaky gut, such as citrus seed extract, berberine and artemesia.

If there are multiple problems, e.g. Candida toxins, over-permeable mucosa, or imbalances in the intestinal flora, these can be corrected by a good therapist, such as a

Kinesiologist, who can test to see exactly what the problems are. Ralph Pike declares,

"The only truly systemic treatment for candida I know of (other than Ketaconozole etc.), is herbal complexes."

Sources for this chapter:-

"Arthritis, the Allergy Connection", by Dr.John Mansfield.
"Maximum Immunity", by Michael A Weiner, Ph.D.
"Candida Albicans", by Stephen Terrass.
"Candida and Thrush", by Dr. George Lewith M.A., M.R.C.P., M.R.C.G.P.
"Candidiasis- an Overview", by R.A.Pike M.R.N.T., K.F.R.P., Dip. MESK.
"Intestinal Permeability", an article by Stephen A. Barrie, ND., and Martin J. Lee , Ph.D.
"Leaky Gut," an article by Leo Gallan, which was printed in "What Doctors don't tell You", August, 1997.

THE DIET FOR CANDIDA

Foods to avoid.

1. Fruits:- all dried fruits, apples, cherries, fresh pine-apple, dark grapes, strawberries, oranges, mangoes, berries, peaches, pears, plums, nectarines.
2. Cereals:- All cereals containing processed sugar.
3. Soups:- All creamy soups, soups with pasta and soups with yeast.
4. Meat, etc.:- All packaged processed meats. Deep fried fish or chicken, fried eggs.

5. Dairy:- All dairy, milk, cheese, yoghourt, cottage cheese, ice-cream, kefir.

6. Vegetables:- Yams, sweet and normal potatoes.

7. Breads:- No commercial breads with yeast, sugar or milk.

8. Drinks:- All alcoholic beverages, diet and regular sodas, undiluted fruit juices, and regular tea or coffee.

9. Desserts:- All desserts made from dairy, refined sugar, honey, maple syrup, artificial sweeteners such as Nutrisweet.

10. Miscellaneous:- All candies and chocolate, jams and jellies, condiments with chemicals, sugar or dairy.

Foods which may be eaten.

1. Fruits:- Grapefruit, Thompson seedless grapes, bananas, cantaloupe, water melon.

(This is debatable. I find that most fruits make my candidiasis symptoms worse.)

2. Cereals:- Wholegrain cereals without sugar.

3. Soups. All broths, miso, vegetable, chicken with vegetable, beef with vegetable.

4. Meat,etc.:- All lean meats, skinless poultry, fish steamed, poached, baked or broiled. Eggs, boiled or poached.

5. Dairy:- None. For cow's milk substitute soya milk or rice milk.

6. Vegetables:-Except for the above mentioned, all others are O.K. unless the person has a sensitivity. Vegetables need to be steamed, baked, boiled, juiced or raw.

7. Breads:- Sprouted grains without yeast or sugar, rice cakes, baked corn chips without fat. Spelt flour bread without yeast, other yeast free breads.

8. Drinks:- Seltzer water, spring water, herb teas, coffee substitutes, diluted fruit juices, (one third juice, two thirds water), Rejuvelac drink, rice milk.

9. Desserts:- All allowable fruits.

10. Miscellaneous:- All soaked raw nuts (peanuts must be roasted). Almond butter, peanut butter and tahini. Mustard, worcestershire sauce, olives, peppers.

One of the most common food intolerances caused by candida is gluten, which is found in wheat, oats, rye and barley. There is no gluten in oatbran or oatgerm. Spelt flour is an excellent substitute for 100% wholemeal flour and can be used to make pasta. Spelt does contain gluten but is well tolerated, -even by coeliacs.

The Candida diet sheet is supplied by Ralph Pike, to whom go my thanks.

APPENDIX 3
THE ARTHRITIC
ASSOCIATION

The Arthritic Association is a voluntary organisation, founded in 1942 in Bournemouth, by a group of people, all of whom had recovered from arthritis.

They had been helped by the methods of the late Charles de Coti Marsh, a rheumatologist and medical scientist, who had successfully been treating arthritis patients since the 1940's. He died in 1968 but his work is continued by the Arthritic Association, now a registered charity. Here is an excerpt from his notes:-

"It must be understood that the disease begins in the bowel. Incorrect diet causes a deficiency of potassium in the blood. The muscles become stiff, cramped and contracted. The joints are drawn closer together and become calcified."

Treatment which people can follow at home aims at recovery by first restoring a good circulation of blood to the muscles. This can be achieved by eating a structured diet of potassium rich foods with the addition of "K" Compound and other supplements, releasing cramped muscles and loosening tight, painful joints. As already mentioned, the remedies and advice I have received have been of great value, contributing enormously to my improvement.

The most fundamental preparation is "K" Compound. The ingredients help to dissolve and disintegrate collections of lime and chalk which lodge within the body. "K" is the chemical symbol for potassium, which is needed by the bloodstream to keep the heart, arteries and blood free from clots and calcification. The use of salt should be restricted when taking "K" Compound as the two are antagonistic.

In diseases such as arthritis the energy level decreases according to the extent of the disease. To help combat this there are Energy Plus tablets, which are composed of natural organic substances. The tablets reinforce natural energy, accelerating improvement and therefore cutting down the time between the stages of recovery. The Detox tablets are advised in cases of sluggish bowel actions; also they are regularly taken on a weekly basis to detoxify the body. These herbal tablets "produce a remedy giving a gentle bowel movement, with no known habit-forming effects." They are especially useful when fasting (- one day a week is recommended by the Association), as they remove the waste matter which accumulates in the colon during a fast.

Other important preparations include Seaweed and Oil of Garlic. Garlic is a natural effective remedy for catarrh, sinusitis and constipation, which are all fore-runners of rheumatoid arthritis. It is rich in vitamins B,C and D, zinc and other minerals; it also purifies the bloodstream and destroys harmful bacteria. Charles de Coti Marsh says: "The author is of the strong opinion that garlic is the most beneficial and natural medicine for both man and animal."

The Deep Seaweed tablets are made from deep oceanic vegetation, rich in minerals and iodine, which is necessary to keep the thyroid gland working properly in balance; a deficiency of iodine causes premature ageing in the body.

The tablets contain normal iodine , also ninety-two supporting trace elements which the gland needs, and other minerals, which are considered to be a nutritional necessity in view of the denaturing of our food caused by the use of chemical fertilisers.

There are many other remedies supplied by the Arthritic Association, including Multivitamin and Mineral tablets, Arnica in place of drugs for the pain, and Rosehip capsules for vitamin C.

The other important substance which is recommended is wheat germ, which is rich in vitamin E. This has excellent energy-giving properties to combat disease, and is described in Charles de Coti Marsh's book, "Prescription for Energy." The fresh untreated wheat should be freshly milled in order to obtain the valuable, energy-giving wheat germ. This is usually taken at breakfast time, but may be added to soups, casseroles etc. The wheat may be ground in a small coffee grinder, which can also be used for grinding nuts, millet and other seeds.

A diet sheet is sent to members which is very easy to follow. Each food is given a points value according to its recommendation for arthritis sufferers, -the "safer" foods have lower points. It is stressed that this is only a guide, of course, as every case is different; some people may react to a particular food while others may not. But it is extremely helpful in that it gives pointers to the foods which are most likely to affect you.

"Home Treatment for Arthritis" is a practical guide designed to help people before and/or after consultation, or for those who cannot attend for a consultation. It includes instructions on how to de-toxify the body before changing to a diet which is rich in potassium, iron and protein, and in energy-giving foods. Suggestions for meals are given.

Special baths are described, and I have found the "hot and cold footbaths" especially helpful, when the knees, feet or ankles have been troublesome.

These consist of having two buckets or bowls of water, one very hot, one cold. Salt, Epsom Salts and iodine are added to each bowl; the instructions for this are given in the book. The feet are placed into the hot water for two minutes and then alternately plunged into the cold and hot water for thirty seconds each. This is repeated for twenty or more alternate plunges.

Also described in the book are the stages of recovery, with details of the remedies to take for each stage.

Useful advice is given on other topics such as clothing, which should be made of natural fibres.

Charles de Coti Marsh was honoured by the French Government for his work with arthritis. His books include:-

Rheumatism and Arthritis- The Conquest.
Prescription for Energy.
Diet for Arthritis.

All of these are obtainable from the Arthritic Association.

Membership of the Association is very reasonable and members receive a free copy of the Home Treatment book, dietary guidance, the all important tablets at reduced prices, the services of a Consultant or therapist for private consultations, and a helpful free magazine, "Rheumatic Review", which is published twice a year.

There is an Annual General Meeting, held in London each April. This includes lunch, which is at a very low price to members.

I have nothing but praise for the Arthritic Association and would strongly recommend anyone with arthritis to join this helpful organisation. (Address at the end of the book.)

BIBLIOGRAPHY, REFERENCES AND FURTHER READING

Primary References

The Art of Changing,by Glen Park; Ashgrove Press,1989.

Arthritis, by Stephen Terrass; Thorsons, 1994.

Arthritis and Rheumatism, by Dr. John Cosh, F.R.C.P. M.D.; Amberwood Publishing Ltd., 1997.

Arthritis, -the Allergy Connection, By Dr. John Mansfield; Thorson's,1990.

Arthritis Cassette Tape, by Stephen Terass; Solgar Vitamins Ltd., Solgar House, Chiltern Commerce Centre, Asheridge Road, Chesham, Bucks. HP5 2PY.

The Arthritis Helpbook, by Kate Lorig and James F. Fries; Souvenir Press,1983.

A Cancer Therapy -Results of Fifty Cases, and The Cure of Advanced Cancer by Diet Therapy, by Max Gerson, M.D.; The Gerson Institute,1958.

Candida Albicans, How Your Diet can Help, by

Stephen Terass; Thorsons, 1996.

Colon Health: The Key to a Vibrant Life, by Norman Walker, D.Sc., Ph.D.; Norwalk Press,1979.

The Complete Raw Juice Therapy; Thorson's Editorial Board.

Detoxification and Healing, by Sidney Macdonald Baker, M.D.; Keats Publishing, Inc., New Canaan, Connecticut, 1997.

Diet for Arthritis, by Charles de Coti-Marsh; Kerbina Ltd. (Obtainable from The Arthritic Association).
Food Combining for Health, by Doris Grant & Jean Joice; Thorson's, 1984.

Food Intolerance and Food Allergy, a Joint Report of the Royal College of Physicians and the British Nutritional Foundation, April 1984.

The Gospel of Peace of Jesus Christ by the Disciple John; C.W.Daniel Co. Ltd., 1937.

A Harmony of Science and Nature, by John and Lucie Davidson; Wholistic Research Co.,1997.

Healing by the Spirit, by Ivan Cooke; published by The White Eagle Publishing Trust, 1980.

How to Beat Inflammation without Drugs, an ION Report on Dr. Jeffrey Bland's Masterclass on Inflammation,
The Institute for Optimum Nutrition, 1997.

An Introduction to the Benefits of tha Bach Flower Remedies, by Jane Evans; The C.W.Daniel Company, 1974.

Living in the Now, by Eckhart Tolle, also The Power of Now, by the same author.

Maximum Immunity, by Michael A. Weiner, Ph.D.; Gateway
Books,1986.

Mucusless Diet Healing System, by Arnold Ehret; Benedict Lust Publications, Box 404, New York, 1970.

Raw Energy, by Leslie & Susannah Kenton; Arrow Books, 1984.

Raw Vegetable Juices, by N.W. Walker; Norwalk Press.

Rheumatism and Arthritis -The Conquest (2nd Edition); Kerbina Ltd. (Obtainable from The Arthritic Association).

Say No to Arthritis, by Patrick Holford; Ion Press, 1993.

Still Here, by Ram Dass.

The Tao of Physics, by Fritjof Capra; Flamingo Books.

Vitamin Guide -Essentials nutrients for Healthy Living, by Hasnain Walji; Element, 1992.

Why Food Allergy, A Report by Patrick Holford; Institute for Optimum Nutrition.

Yoga for You, by Indra Devi; Harper Collins Publishers. First published by Thorsons,1960.

You Can Heal Your Life, by Louise Hay; Eden Grove Editions, 1987.

Other References and Further Reading

Aloe Vera, the Natural Healer, by Paul Hornsey-Pennell, published by The Wordsmith Publishing Company, 1994.

Alternative Medicine, A Guide to Natural Therapies, by Dr. Andrew Stanway, published by Bloomsbury Books, London,1992.

The Causation of Rheumatoid Disease and Many Human Cancers: A New Concept in Medicine, by Roger Wynburn-Mason; Tokyo, Iji Publishing Company, 1978.

The Celestine Prophecy, by James Redfield. Bantam Books,1994.

E for Additives, by Maurice Hanssen; Thorson's,1984.

Emotional & personality factors in the onset and course of autoimmune disease, particularly rheumatoid arthritis, by

Dr. G.F. Solomon, in Psychoneuroimmunology; Ader,R., ed., Academic Press, N.Y.

A Handbook for Light Workers, by David Cousins; Barton House Publishing, Bath, BA1 2XJ, 1993.

Hands of Light, -A Guide to Healing through the Human Energy Field, by Barbara Ann Brennan; Bantam Books, 1987.

Light Emerging, by Barbara Ann Brennan; Bantam Books, 1993.

Love Your Disease, by John Harrison; Angus & Robertson Publishers, London, 1984.

The Massage Book, by George Downing; Penguin, 1974.

The Medical Discoveries of Edward Bach, Physician, by Norah Weeks; C.W.Daniel & Co. Ltd.

Peace Pilgrim, Compiled by some of her friends; An Ocean Tree Book, Santa Fe, New Mexico, 1994.

Prescription for Energy, by Charles de Coti-Marsh; Kerbina Ltd. (Obtainable form The Arthritic Association).

The Prophet, by Khalil Gibran; William Heinemann Ltd., 1972.

The Quiet Mind, published by The White Eagle Publishing Trust.

Shiatsu -Japanese Massage for Health & Fitness, by Elaine Liechti; Element Books, 1992.

The Silent Path,by Michael J. Eastcott; Rider Books.

Uninvited Guests, by Hermann Bueno, M.D., published by Keats Publishing, Inc.

Subtle Energy, by John Davidson; C.W.Daniel Co. Ltd., 1987.

Tao -The Watercourse Way, by Alan Watts; Arkana, Penguin Books.

The Wave, Ecstatic Dance for Body & Soul; (Video). Raven Recording, P. O. Box 2034, Red Bank NJ 07701, 201-642, 1979, U.S.A.

Ask your Angels, by Wyllie, Daniel & Ramer; Ballantine Books, New York,1992.

Budo Chi, A Martial Arts Way of Healing and Strengthening. Video by Mark A. Newns.

ACKNOWLEDGEMENTS

Grateful thanks to the following publishers, authors and healing practitioners for permission to use quotations:-

Author House, for all their help.
The Quiet Mind, Healing by the Spirit, and the calendar by permission of the White Eagle Publishing Trust, New Lands, Liss, Hampshire, United Kingdom.
The Arthritic Association.
David Cousins.
Harper Collins Publishers.
Dr. John Mansfield.
Ralph A. Pike, M.R.N.T., K.F.R.P., Dip. M.E.S.K.
Glen Park
John Davidson, Wholistic Research Co.

I would also like to acknowledge the help of various friends and practitioners who have helped by reading various chapters and offering invaluable advice.

Brian Hampton, Nutritionist, The Caring Clinic, Sheffield.
Dr. K.L. Jensen, Chiropractor.
Ralph Pike, Kinesiologist. Nature's Trail, Sheffield.
Jerry Shevills, Sheffield School of Massage.
David Keith.
Ray Tubbs.

A special thank you goes to Nick Mason, my computor guide and rescuer, for his unfailing patience. Without his help writing this book would have proved a formidable task.

ADDRESSES

The Arthritic Association,
First Floor Suite,
2, Hyde Gardens,,
Eastbourne,
East Sussex,
BN21 4PN.

Alexander Technique
20, London House,
London ,
SW 10 9EL. Tel: 0171 351 0828.

Arthritis Care,
18 Stephenson Way,
London,
NW1 2HD. Tel: 0171 916 1500
Free Help Line 0800 289 170
(Mon-Fri. 12-4p.m.)

The British Chiropractic Association
5 First Avenue,
Chelmsford,
Essex,
CM1 1RX.

The British Herbal Medicine Association,
Field House,

Lye Hole Lane,
Redhill,
Avon,
BS18 7TB.

The British Homoeopathic Association,
27A Devonshire Street,
London,
W1N 1RJ. Tel: 0171 935 2163.

The British Naturapathic and Osteopathic Association,
6 Netherhall Gardens,
London,
NW3 5RR.
Tel: 0171 435 8728.

The British Shiatsu Association,
Townsend House,
Wolverley,
Kidderminster,
Worcester,
DY11 5XF.

Higher Nature,
The Nutrition Centre,
Burwash Common,
East Sussex.
TN19 7LX.
Tel: 0435 883484.

Individual Diet Company,
The Old Mill,
The Street,
Albury, Surrey.
GU5 9AZ.
Tel: 0483 203555

Institute for Optimum Nutrition,
Blades Court,
Deodar Road,
London,
SW15 2NU.

Christina Lausevic, Kinesiologist,
60, Sidney Grove,
Newcastle-on- Tyne.
NE4 5PD.
Tel: 01912411963

The National Federation of Spiritual Healers,
Old Manor Farm Studio,
Church Street,
Sunbury-on-Thames,
Middlesex,
TW16 6RG.

National Institute of Medical Herbalists,
Hon General Secretary,
56 Longbrook Street,
Exeter,
Devon,
EX4 6AH.

Northern School of Reflexology,
32, Handsworth Gardens,
Doncaster,
DN3 3SZ.

Parascope Laboratory,
Department of Microbiology,
Chapel Allerton Hospital,
Chapeltown Road,
Leeds.
LS7 4SA.

White Eagle Lodge,
New Lands,
Brewells Lane,
Liss, Hants,
GU33 7HY.

York Nutritional Laboratory,
Tudor House,
Lysander Close,
Clifton Moor,
York.
YO3 4XB.
Tel: 0904 690640